When the Music Stopped

My Battle and Victory against MS

Bob Cafaro

Bob Cafaro, LLC
Website: www.bobcafaro.com
Email: info@bobcafaro.com

Cafaro, Bob.
When the Music Stopped: My Battle and Victory against MS /
Bob Cafaro. – 1st ed., 2nd printing.

ISBN 978-0-9971432-1-8

Reviews for *When the Music Stopped*

"If you are ever presented with something that seems impossible to defeat, reading Bob's book will give you the strength and inspiration to create your own miracle and escape from that dark night. It could be an illness, a financial issue or even a relationship failure. This book will inspire you, as it has inspired me."

-Nando Parrado
Survivor, and Author of Miracle in the Andes

"Bob Cafaro and his story should be a must read for patients, families, caregivers, and physicians and surgeons who face the devastation of punishing chronic diseases. Through his courage and resolve, Bob overcame multiple sclerosis, one of the most punishing of all diseases. This book chronicles in riveting detail how this world class cellist for The Philadelphia Orchestra delivered his best personal medical performance.
Ironically, during the time when I first met Bob, my wife and I had watched the movie "Hilary and Jackie," the tragic saga of Jacqueline du Pré, the internationally known cellist whose life had been cut short by MS.
As I tried to counsel and console Bob, my mind was obsessed with the thought that he had known the heart-rending story of another cellist afflicted by MS. We offered Bob compassion, sympathy, and some glimmer of hope. As his book reveals, Bob did the rest.
His courage is an improbable combination of the pure determination of Rocky ascending the steps of the Philadelphia Museum of Art and the beauty and grace of du Pré's famous performance of Elgar's Cello Concerto."

-Robert C. Sergott, MD
Director of Neuro-Ophthalmology, Wills Eye Hospital, Philadelphia, PA

"Authentic, honest, moving and inspiring... This story is an invaluable lesson for those who love music, health, and life."

-Yannick Nézet Séguin
Conductor and Music Director of The Philadelphia Orchestra

"This poignant and powerful memoir recounts the story of Bob Cafaro, a gifted cellist who was stricken with multiple sclerosis in the prime of his life. Rather than succumb to a disease that was voraciously eating his nervous system and robbing him of even the most basic human functions, Mr. Cafaro chose to fight back. Through a combination of sheer tenacity and uncanny street-sense, he was able to devise a multifaceted approach to overcoming an illness that appeared to be his death sentence. Arming himself with a unique mixture of modern medical therapies, radical changes in diet, exercise, and mental focus, Mr. Cafaro beat the odds. A decade and a half ago his brain and spinal cord were riddled with incapacitating lesions. He was left virtually blind, had profound weakness and numbness, and could not even lift a pen to write his own epitaph. Today he is symptom free and enjoying his life as a member of one of the greatest orchestras in the world, the Philadelphia Orchestra. Mr. Cafaro stresses that his formula worked for him, and it may not be applicable to others suffering from the disease. His 'shotgun' approach, targeting his enemy from every angle imaginable, led to what was and perhaps is considered to be a medical impossibility – the eradication of MS from the body. Perhaps out of the myriad of 'bullets' only a few or even one had the firepower to eliminate the villain. But it doesn't really matter. He is alive and well and has graciously shared his story for others to be inspired and to never give up the battle, or hope. A must read!"

-Eric Roter, M.D.
Attending Physician, Metro Hospital, Cleveland, OH

"Bob Cafaro, cellist in the world-renowned Philadelphia Orchestra, in his memoir When the Music Stopped: My Battle and Victory against MS, recounts the astounding story of how he cured himself of multiple sclerosis. With humor and passion, he details his journey from "on top of the world," to the depths of disease and despair, back to the peak of health, where he remains to this day. He includes a veritable primer on the unconventional weapons he wielded in his fight to regain his life: hydration, diet, exercise, and meditation.

As a physician, musician, and Philadelphian, I found this book to be especially captivating, but it will resonate with any person whose life has been directly or indirectly affected by MS or a similarly devastating illness. I look forward to recommending it to others, including my patients, as a much-needed ray of hope in the face of what can often appear to be a hopeless condition."

Karen Fung Dante, M.D.
Classical singer and Associate Surgeon, Wills Eye Hospital, Philadelphia, PA

Five Stars
"I was diagnosed with MS a year ago, I found Bob Cafaro's book full of valuable information and inspiration."

Five Stars
"Great writer, teacher. If you are searching for inspiration and perseverance herein lies a terrific role model."

Five Stars
"So much positivity! To learn through others, and learn how to apply methods to help in your life..."

Five Stars
"Wow!! An amazing book! Such a "page turner." Riveting … This is a must read."

Five Stars
"Just what I needed. An inspiration while going through a challenging time. Thank you!"

-Amazon Customer Reviews

This book is dedicated to everyone who battles MS day-in and day-out. Never give up searching for that light which is shining brightly at the end of the tunnel.

To my mother, Kit, and my wife, Teresa.

I wish to express my sincerest gratitude to the following people. It would not have been possible to write this book without their invaluable wisdom, advice and assistance:

Tyler Willis

Tammy Brenn

LeeAnne Hogan

Nando Parrado

Dan Fernando

Diana Regan

Tony Gizzi

Steve Zvengrowski

Jane Zvengrowski

Dorothea Courtwright

Eleanor Pollak

Jessica Griffin

Dawn Williams

Jack and Eve Kenyon

One very special and passionate couple who wishes to remain anonymous

Contents

Disclaimer

It is important to note that this book is not a cure for any illness or disease.

The steps the author has followed to fight Multiple Sclerosis (MS) are for informational purposes only and they are not a promise or a guarantee of any result. Before following any of the steps outlined in this book, readers are advised to conduct their own research and consult with their own medical professionals.

Prologue

Prelude to an Early Ending

It was the 16th day of August 1999. Five days earlier, I was released from the hospital where I spent four days for extreme motion sickness and severe dehydration. The motion sickness was not the result of any motion, but it was one of several effects of my third and most vicious Multiple Sclerosis (MS) attacks to date. The dehydration resulted from several days of persistent vomiting and an inability to retain any food or water. My previous two MS attacks were child's play compared to this latest one, and I was now dealing with something far more formidable and ruthless. Since my first symptoms eight months earlier I worked hard to convince myself that MS was a misdiagnosis but it was now time to face up to the hard ugly truth. Now I was barely able to walk and unable to drive due to a partial loss of vision in both eyes, and the use of my hands was severely impaired as my entire central nervous system had gone haywire. The lines of communication from the brain to many parts of my body were cut off. To make things worse, I was now partially incontinent. This latest attack mainly targeted the eyes and hands, which is a devastating combination for a professional cellist. Being home after the hospital stay was a relief as the four days spent lying in a hospital bed felt like I was trapped in a coffin.

Needing some sunshine in my life, I took my cello out of the case to make sure I could still play. When a person does something on a regular basis for most of their life it becomes second nature. When I proceeded to tune the cello, it was an unexpected shock to find that simply drawing the bow across the strings with my right arm was nearly impossible. The left hand was even worse as I was unable to line up four fingers on one string. After a few minutes of trying to get settled, I attempted playing the Prelude to the Suite No. 1 for Unaccompanied Cello by Johann Sebastian Bach. This is a piece I know very well as I studied it as a child and performed it countless times. What took place next was one of the worst experiences of my life. I knew what to do and how to do it but the result was like a five-year-old child learning how to play the cello with little understanding of how to go about it. It was a horrible feeling and the sound that was coming from the cello was even worse.

After several unsuccessful and utterly hopeless lines of Bach, I cleaned off the cello and placed it back in its case. Then I dropped to my knees and began to cry like a child. Everything in life that I had taken for granted had now been stripped away. Not only was it impossible to play the cello but I could no longer write legibly or even hold a phone without dropping it. In addition to losing control of my fingers, both hands were left with almost no feeling. They had a "pins and needles" feeling as if they had fallen asleep from loss of circulation. Even simple tasks such as holding money or paper were now a challenge because there was no way of knowing if something slipped out of my hand. For the first time I seriously contemplated ending my misery as I did not want to live this way or be a burden to my children. In just eight short months, MS had transformed my dream life to a life in hell.

-Part I-

Chapter 1

The Dream Life

My childhood would be considered ordinary when compared to most kids, but it was different from the childhoods of most professional classical musicians. As one of four children, I grew up in a single income household where my father worked for several different companies, and we lived on his modest income that was sufficient to just make ends meet. Neither of my parents played an instrument and classical music was not part of the household culture. My dad was clever in many ways, and he was always on the lookout for ways to stretch a buck and find ways to ethically beat the system. His philosophy of life was anything but ordinary; the seeds he planted in the hearts and minds of his children later blossomed into fruit bearing trees. After high school my father attended college for two years where he received his associate degree in mechanical engineering. After my mother finished high school she attended secretarial school and then devoted herself to raising four children. When I was young my father started a business with my Uncle Jack who was a volunteer firefighter, and together they came up with some clever and needed inventions for fire trucks and firefighters. With the aid of his mechanical engineering background, my dad invented an automatic water-powered hose winder that cleaned and rolled up the long heavy hoses after a fire was extinguished. Uncle Jack's field of expertise was electrical engineering, and he invented an electronic water meter, which indicated the water level in the tank of the fire truck. The big advantage of this revolutionary water meter was the four bright red lights that were on the side panel of the fire truck. Firefighters were now able to see the lights and know the water level from a distance. After several years of working together, my father and Uncle Jack went separate ways to independently pursue their own business opportunities. In their new business endeavors, they mutually agreed to swap inventions, so Uncle Jack would keep the hose winder and my dad kept the water meter. Both of them went on to establish successful small businesses, and they later put all their children through college without the burden of student loans.

When I was in third grade in public school at the age of nine, all students in my school were required to take a general music class. Everyone in the class was given a musical aptitude test, and I apparently scored well on the exam. I remember clowning around with the answers and seeing my feeble attempts at humor marked with big red X's by the teacher. The music teacher must have known she was dealing with a frustrated future comedian with musical talent, because I brought home a letter stating I had been selected to begin learning to play a string instrument. Back then, I was suffering with childhood asthma, and I wanted to play the trumpet because it might somehow have therapeutic value for my lungs. At my first meeting with the elementary school string teacher Dorothy Bennert, I asked for her opinion on the matter and she said playing the trumpet would make no difference with asthma. Learning the trumpet would have meant a one-year delay because the students were not allowed to play a brass instrument until the fourth grade. Mrs. Bennert then used her persuasive powers to convince me to forego the trumpet and immediately begin a string instrument. After quickly settling that matter the next step was to decide which string instrument I would play. The choice was the violin, viola, cello or bass, and since there was no musical background in my family, I barely knew the difference between the instruments. At that point, Mrs. Bennert took the initiative and explained that there was no one to play cello in the elementary school orchestra. She said I could play any string instrument I wanted – as long as it was the cello. After a moment of thought, I told Mrs. Bennert I wanted to play the cello, and she smiled approvingly at my wise choice.

And so my life as a cellist commenced at the comparatively late age of nine. The initial draw to the cello was magical, and that was no doubt largely due to my mother's proud and smiling face every time I played. One year after starting the instrument, I was featured as soloist at one of the elementary school orchestra concerts. Mrs. Bennert, the string teacher, was impressed that I had taught myself the skill of vibrating on the cello with the left hand. That led to my renowned solo cello debut at the concert. The two pieces I played were the popular songs *More* and *Love is Blue*. My mother glowed throughout my performance and I still remember her smile that night. Unfortunately, my non-musical life at home did not help to sustain my interest in the cello. As time progressed, the instrument became a target of ridicule by other kids and I quickly lost interest. As fear and self-consciousness began to take hold, I became resentful of the cello and wanted to quit. To make matters worse, the friends I spent time with growing up were a negative influence. It is often possible to look at a child and promptly determine if they are destined for greatness or a life of trouble. Two of my friends in particular had the latter path in their future, and they headed down their respective, troubled roads in overdrive. One had a bad LSD experience in his teens. He was brought home from a rock concert by the police, and his life continued in the wrong direction. He later wound up in prison for burglary. My other friend also had his first brush with the law when he was in his teens. He was arrested and taken away in handcuffs at a local restaurant for stealing a two-dollar tip off one of the tables. This one later burglarized a veterinarian's office and stole a large quantity of unknown drugs. From his ill-gotten gains, he swallowed two pills without knowing their purpose. The pills were used to euthanize animals, and tragically his life was cut short.

Fortunately, I was scared away from these acquaintances when they turned to drugs and crime. Many of their peers considered them "cool" at the time, but they would now make interesting subjects in one of those "Where are they now?" articles.

Planning my Future

The first time my parents required the services of an attorney, my father was aghast when he received an itemized invoice of the firm's billable hours. From that moment, he wanted all of his children to become lawyers to ensure they would enjoy a prosperous future. My older brother and sister fulfilled his expectations and became successful attorneys, but my younger sister and I did not. Since I am the sole musician in the family, I seriously considered living up to Dad's expectations by specializing in the field of music malpractice.

I feel so fortunate to have inherited the best traits of both my parents. My father was very street-smart and his mechanical intuition gave him an advantage when it came to figuring out how to do things. My mother is truly a good soul and one of the most generous people I have ever known. One childhood memory that always remained with me describes my mother's human side. In the early 1960's, our family went to the drive-in theater to see the newly released movie *The Sound of Music*. I was very young and remember little from the movie, but I can still see my mother in the front seat crying during the film. That was the first time I remember seeing my mother cry. Even though it was during a movie, I have never stopped trying to understand why my mother was crying in that moment. There is little doubt I inherited this particular trait from Mom because I always cry during movies.

On Top of the World

In December of 1998, I was on top of the world. Ever since 1985 I have been a cellist with the Philadelphia Orchestra, which is truly one of the greatest orchestras in the world. Becoming a member of such an esteemed ensemble is no easy feat. When I auditioned for the Philadelphia position, there were 149 other cellists competing for the one opening. Countless disciplined hours of daily work over many years are required to win an audition that is about twenty minutes in length. Musicians competing for major orchestra openings are no different from athletes competing for an Olympic gold medal. The slightest mistake or momentary lapse in Olympic competition will make a judge's decision easier, and it will cost a competitor a medal. Competing for a major orchestra position is brutally similar because flawless instrumental playing is required to win an audition.

In addition to being a member of the Philadelphia Orchestra, my cello teaching was equally successful. I had several fine cello students, and I was teaching cello and coaching ensembles at the Hartwick Summer Music Festival in Oneonta, NY every summer since 1987.

At age forty, I was in excellent physical condition with almost no visible body fat. Since my teen years, every morning began with a yoga session and most days I biked the seven miles to and from the train station for my commute to work with the orchestra. I lived on a diet largely void of processed food and did not smoke, drink or take recreational drugs. Living this way instilled every confidence that becoming a centenarian was in my future and I would certainly never face any serious illness before that 100-year landmark.

My Introduction to Multiple Sclerosis

In December of 1998, I saw the movie *Hilary and Jackie*, the biography of the great British cellist Jacqueline du Pré whose brilliant career and life were tragically cut short by MS. She was a regular guest soloist with the world's greatest orchestras, including the Philadelphia Orchestra. Several of my senior colleagues who were in the orchestra when Jacqueline du Pré appeared, talk about what a unique and brightly shining light she was. Jacqueline du Pré was a truly extraordinary cellist and many of her recordings including those with Philadelphia, are a testament to her exceptional artistry. MS forced Jacqueline du Pré to stop playing the cello at the age of twenty-six, and she passed away from MS-related complications at the age of forty-two.

MS is a mysterious neurological disorder that is different from many other diseases. The disease was discovered and named in 1868 by the French neurologist Jean Martin Charcot. There is no blood test for MS; it is diagnosed by a process of elimination. Diagnosing the disease is often a lengthy and frustrating ordeal and the anxiety before and after a diagnosis is sometimes worse than the diagnosis itself. MS is a disorder of the body's immune system, which for unknown reasons attacks the central nervous system. Women are diagnosed with MS more than men by at least a 2 to 1 margin and the disease is most common in people age 20 – 50.

The nerves and the nerve fibers of the central nervous system are protected by a fatty myelin sheath and MS causes the immune system to attack and destroy the myelin as well as the nerves and nerve fibers. The damaged myelin leaves behind scar tissue; this scar tissue is otherwise known as 'sclerosis.' This damage to the myelin, the nerves, and the nerve fibers affects the ability of the brain to transmit signals to the body. In my particular case the progression of MS had a snowball effect because it gained in size and strength as time progressed and my health deteriorated.

About one week after seeing *Hilary and Jackie*, a strange numbness appeared in my right leg, and it was different from any numbness I had ever experienced. Initially, I was not worried but after one week the numbness progressed to a point of concern. During the time of this mysterious numbness, the Philadelphia Orchestra visited the Kennedy Center in Washington, D.C. for its annual subscription concert. At the conclusion of the dress rehearsal before the concert I stepped down from the stage riser onto the stage, and my right leg collapsed from under me. Luckily, I managed to avoid falling and smashing my cello. This was now a serious situation that clearly warranted medical attention. From the backstage house phone, I was able to schedule appointments with two doctors. The first was with my orthopedic surgeon in Philadelphia, PA, and the second was with my primary care doctor in Cherry Hill, NJ.

After examining my leg, my orthopedist said the condition did not seem serious and was likely a pinched nerve. Several days later when I saw my primary care doctor, he agreed with the probable pinched nerve diagnosis and concurred that there was no need to worry. Before visiting my primary care doctor I looked up my symptoms in the *Mayo Clinic Health Book*, and there were indications my condition pointed to possible early signs of MS. This possibility was brought up with my family doctor who comforted me with words of assurance: "My wife has MS and I know the disease well. What you have is definitely not MS." It was a relief to hear those words from a medical doctor who had firsthand experience with the disease. As one can imagine there had been some understandable anxiety from what I had read in the *Mayo Clinic Health Book.*

Over the next few weeks, the numbness in my right leg gradually disappeared, but strange blood blisters began appearing on the toes of both feet. The blood blisters lasted only a few weeks but they left purple colored scars that remained visible for several months.

Chapter 2

Keeping an Eye Out for Me

By late January 1999, the numbness in the right leg was completely gone, the blood blisters on the toes were clearing up and everything seemed to be returning to normal. Then one month later in February of 1999 I was hit with a sudden loss of vision in my left eye. The initial symptoms seemed like a simple case of dry eye, but after constantly comparing the vision in both eyes, it was clear this was an actual loss of vision. It was not a total vision loss as if the eye was covered with a patch, but actual areas of vision had strangely disappeared from view.

The *Mayo Clinic Health Book* said it was now time to see a neurologist. I did not know any neurologists, as there was never a need for one in the past. For an appointment, I called several neurologists listed in the *Blue Cross Personal Choice Provider* book, but they were all booked in advance for several weeks. After several hours on the phone, I was able to get an appointment with a neurosurgeon in Philadelphia who took me right away I had only one visit with this elderly neurosurgeon. After listening to the history of the recent numbness in my right leg, he examined my optic nerve, which can be partially seen through the pupil of the eye with the use of an ophthalmoscope. This neurosurgeon was a gentle person but a terrible liar because his facial expression was unable to hide what he was thinking. There was little doubt as to what was on his mind and without saying what was wrong he stressed the importance of seeing a neurologist immediately. I pressed him for a diagnosis but he invoked the Fifth Amendment and remained silent. With no hint of a diagnosis, he set up an appointment with Dr. Michael Robert Sperling, a neurologist with Jefferson Hospital in Philadelphia, PA, who is known for his expertise in epilepsy.

The First Neurologist - Dr. Michael Sperling

There was a one-week wait for the appointment with Dr. Sperling, and that waiting time gave the MS ample time to continue its work on the optic nerve of my left eye. When I finally saw Dr. Sperling, he ordered an immediate MRI of the brain, which is standard procedure for a patient with my symptoms. MRI technology in 1999 was primitive compared to the instant digital imagery technology of today. At the following visit, Dr. Sperling fastened the antiquated oversized film sheets of my brain onto the backlit screen and he guided me through the basics of an MRI of the brain. He pointed out there were no visible lesions present, and I breathed a huge sigh of relief that it was not MS. Then he told me straight out: "You have MS." I stared at him in a complete state of shock because the only thing I knew about MS was Jacqueline du Pré and her exceptionally horrible case of the disease. With the combination of the numbness in the right leg and the loss of vision in the left eye, I had growing suspicions it was MS. When a respected neurologist actually said I had the disease, I was devastated.

Seeing that I was clearly upset, Dr. Sperling calmly said there was nothing to worry about. He reassuringly continued by saying, "Many people with MS live an absolutely normal life and about half of the people who have MS will never know it." When asked how it was possible to have MS without any lesions in the brain, he said it was not only possible but also common. I continued voicing my doubts, asking if a 40-year-old male was a little old to be getting MS and he told of his recent MS diagnosis of a 53-year-old male. However, I was unable to accept his diagnosis because the clean MRI of the brain said otherwise. *I* knew better. Unfortunately, this was my last visit with Dr. Sperling, whom I consider an excellent neurologist.

This was a classic case of "shooting the messenger" because I was emotionally unable to handle such a diagnosis. Desperate for a different opinion, I came up with a myriad of reasons why he was mistaken. In my state of denial, I even reasoned that because Dr. Sperling was an epilepsy specialist, his knowledge and experience with MS had to be limited. In retrospect, it may have been a wise decision to stay with Dr. Sperling because of his excellent bedside manners, his calm demeanor and his view that MS is a very manageable disease. He was also a subscriber to the Philadelphia Orchestra, and that would have no doubt been advantageous later that summer. Accepting his diagnosis back then was not even a remote possibility, and it would be some time before I was forced to come to terms with it. Unfortunate events would take place in the coming months that I would need to see for myself.

Several months after that last visit with Dr. Sperling, he happened to come to a Philadelphia Orchestra concert at the Academy of Music, which was the orchestra's former home before moving to The Kimmel Center. During the intermission of the concert we ran into each other in the congregating area that is known as the Green Room, and he asked how things were going. At this point, my symptoms had cleared up and instead of a definitive diagnosis, I had been placed in the 'high probability' category for MS by the neurologist Dr. Fred Lublin. I told Dr. Sperling that MS was a misdiagnosis. With the look of a non-believer he explained how the combined symptoms of numbness in one leg and vision loss in one eye "are a textbook case of MS." He asked me to send him my current medical records, but I was so busy hanging on to the hope of a misdiagnosis that I had no desire to have a neurologist second-guessing my misdiagnosis mindset. I never sent him any of the records and it was the last time we saw each other.

The First Visit with Neuro-Ophthalmologist Dr. Robert Sergott

Because of the vision loss in my left eye, Dr. Sperling promptly sent me to Wills Eye Hospital in Philadelphia, where I had my first of many visits with the neuro-ophthalmologist Dr. Robert Sergott. After administering a basic vision test, a visual field test and examining the affected optic nerve, Dr. Sergott explained that the loss of vision in the left eye was a condition known as optic neuritis. A person can never fully understand optic neuritis from a description, from studying the condition in a medical book, or even from firsthand experience in a medical practice. One must actually experience the condition for a true understanding.

One analogy of the condition is with a lamp that is plugged into an electrical outlet. If the electrical cord to the lamp is faulty, the light bulb will flicker and fail to produce a steady light. Another analogy is a television set that gets poor reception. The television functions correctly and the signal is being transmitted, but interference is present and the television does not receive a complete signal, resulting in an incomplete and grainy picture on the screen. Think of the eye as the transmitter of the signal and the brain as the receiver. The brain receives an incomplete signal due to a faulty transmission by the optic nerve, and the visual picture is incomplete. These are the best analogies I was able to come up with after countless unsuccessful attempts at explaining optic neuritis to people. The optic nerve is an extremely complex wonder that is made up of over 1,000,000 layers, and without a second thought it is expected to work perfectly at all times.

After Dr. Sergott's explanation of optic neuritis, he prescribed the standard steroid treatment of 1000 mg of intravenous (IV) methylprednisolone every day for three days to calm the inflammation of the optic nerve. The intravenous steroid treatment would be followed up with oral prednisone, beginning at 100 mg per day, and gradually tapering off to finish at 10 mg per day. To illustrate the potency of 1000 mg of intravenous methylprednisolone, consider one standard prednisone tablet is 20 mg. Therefore 1000 mg of methylprednisolone is equivalent to 1,250 mg of prednisone, or imagine swallowing 62.5 prednisone tablets.

Dr. Sergott did not suspect any misdiagnosis. Since MS is his area of expertise and he is considered one of the very best in his field, I left his office feeling the entire MS drama was a nightmare from which I would soon awaken. I kept telling myself none of this was happening and the entire episode was one big mistake. Having MS was just not possible. This disease only affects other people.

Chapter 3

The Dream

The initial anxiety of dealing with MS day and night is emotionally exhausting and it was consuming more of my life each day. After arriving home from the office visit with Dr. Sperling, it was still the middle of the day, but I promptly crawled into bed and fell into a deep sleep. The bad news of my diagnosis ruled out any restful sleep and I had a disturbing dream that was a replay of a childhood experience many years earlier.

In 1961 when I was three, my family moved from a row house in Queens, New York City, to a newly built house in Smithtown, New York, which is on Long Island, fifty miles east of Manhattan. The entire area was being newly developed and our house was only the second one built on the entire block. To illustrate just how new the place was, the main access route Veterans Memorial Highway, which is currently a heavily travelled six-lane highway complete with jammed traffic much of the day, had not even been paved yet. This area was so rural that my grandfather questioned the wisdom of my parents' move to such a remote location, and he referred to it as "the asshole of the world." Our new house had a huge backyard that extended deep into the woods, and about twenty-five yards into the heavy brush the builders dug a shallow pit where they thoughtlessly disposed of various unwanted building materials. The discarded items ranged from asbestos shingles to five-gallon metal buckets of glues, sealants, and other chemicals. It was an incredibly quiet and secluded place and as a child I often went there for solitary playtime, withdrawing into my own imaginary world for hours at a time.

In the dream I went back in time to my childhood where everything was just as I remembered. There wasn't a cloud in the sky and I was sitting in the pit playing with all the discarded building materials and buckets just as I had done as a child. I awoke from the dream startled and wondered if there was any correlation between this childhood experience in the pit and my diagnosis of MS thirty-five years later. Since childhood I had not thought of the time playing there, but this dream hit like a bolt from the blue and with incredibly vivid reality. Since that dream I have been wondering about possible long-term health effects on children when they are exposed to chemicals such as solvents and sealants. Could my exposure to those chemicals be linked to my diagnosis of MS more than 30 years later?

Later that evening I was so depressed that I downed three glasses of wine. Because my system had never built up a tolerance for alcohol, the unnatural substance made my head spin. I never drank much because the acquired taste for alcohol is something I had never learned. My first drinking experience was intended as a rite of passage, but instead it turned out to be an event that put a stop to serious drinking for the rest of my life.

My initiation into the world of alcohol took place when I was in seventh grade while my parents were away on vacation. My brother Billy, who is four years older, had some of his drinking buddies over for a party and they were all getting inebriated. With the energetic enthusiasm of a puppy, I wanted to get drunk and earn my early membership into this club. So, my brother expertly guided me through the intricacies of raiding Dad's liquor cabinet by siphoning small amounts from each bottle to conceal the pilfering of his stash. After forcing down gulp after gulp of wine, scotch, rum and ouzo, my head began to spin and an unexpected nausea set in. Then I ran to the bathroom and vomited violently as my body repeatedly convulsed to rid itself of the poisonous mix. When there was nothing left to vomit, I got into bed and laid there with my head spinning, feeling like I was stuck on some sickening amusement park ride. The next morning I was greeted with a pounding headache from a hangover, which is a feeling a child definitely should not experience.

Staying home sick was not an option so I bit the bullet and boarded the school bus for the forty-five-minute ride to school. The ride on the bus only worsened the hangover and motion sickness was now added to the headache, so the entire ride to school was a struggle to keep from vomiting on the bus. I managed to make it to school without embarrassing myself on the bus, but I felt sick and nauseous for the remainder of the day. There was no choice but to tough it out because going to the school nurse would no doubt have revealed the cause of my condition.

My brother intended the previous evening of drinking as an initiation into the drinking world, but I learned all too well where the word intoxication comes from. Alcohol, like tobacco or spicy food, is an acquired taste that we not only learn to tolerate, but also learn to enjoy. Give an infant a fine Bordeaux wine or a good Cuban cigar, and they will choke on it, spit it out, then cry and scream.

Speaking of Cuban cigars, my one and only experience with them was after my trip to Havana, Cuba, in 1980. During my senior year at Juilliard, I played in a trio. We were invited to play on Holland America Cruise Line's S.S. Rotterdam for twenty-eight days of a 100-day round the world cruise. After a 17-½ hour flight from Kennedy Airport in New York to Cape Town, South Africa, I boarded the cruise ship that had sailed from New York two months earlier. After setting sail from Cape Town, that old sensation of nausea set in while I was seated at dinner, and thus began a journey of seasickness that accompanied me for the remainder of the twenty-eight-day cruise.

There were several celebrities on the ship and among them was the late astronaut Wally Schirra. I got to know him and he was kind enough to give me some advice on remedies that helped him with motion sickness in space. Having suffered from the same symptoms in space, he advised using marezine instead of Dramamine® due to the lesser side effect of drowsiness.

After crossing the Atlantic Ocean and sailing up the coast of South America, the ship stopped in Havana, Cuba, and I was able to get genuine Partagas cigars for $15.50 for a box of 25 cigars. This was an opportunity of a lifetime so I proceeded to roll the dice and smuggle seven boxes of these genuine smokes in my luggage. The trip through customs went like clockwork and I got through without attracting any attention or being searched. After arriving home with the contraband, six boxes of the cigars were given out as gifts and the last box was given out as individual cigars.

From the perspective of a non-smoker, it was intriguing how people could be so ecstatic to receive genuine Cuban cigars that were personally smuggled into the country, so I had to try one. Sitting out on my front porch, I lit one up and began puffing away. These were the best cigars in the world, and because the taste was rather unpleasant, I was certainly missing something. There was little doubt that continued puffing would soon reveal the magic of those wonderful Havana cigars. After smoking about one-third of the cigar and feeling slightly nauseous, I extinguished the stogie and went into the bathroom. A look in the mirror showed my face was now a curious shade of green, then without warning vomiting commenced with a vengeance. As I kneeled over hugging the rim of the toilet, my body struggled to expel the poisons of the world's finest tobacco. With a horrible taste of vomit and cigar juice in my mouth and nose, the only thought going through my mind was, "How could anyone possibly like Cuban cigars?"

Following the celebration of my diagnosis with three glasses of wine, I took advantage of the situation and decided since I had never acquired a taste for alcohol, it would be placed out at the curb on trash day for good. That was February 1999 and it was my last drink of alcohol.

Chapter 4

Intravenous Steroids

After returning home from that first visit with Dr. Sergott at Wills Eye Hospital, I made the phone call to immediately begin intravenous steroids. The next day a traveling nurse visited me, and she brought all the paraphernalia needed to initiate the steroid drip. She began the process by inserting a catheter into a vein on my hand where it remained for the following three days. She hooked up a gravity-fed IV drip of methylprednisolone and the powerful dose began to flow into my body. Methylprednisolone is a steroid that prevents the release of substances in the body that cause inflammation. After finishing three days on intravenous steroids, it was tapered down with six weeks of oral prednisone.

Looking back on this first treatment of steroids, it did stabilize the vision loss but I believe the one-week delay in beginning this treatment was costly. To take stock at this point, the numbness in my left leg had completely cleared up, but the vision in my left eye had not returned to normal. My left eye had a small permanent and bothersome peripheral vision loss as well as some mild loss of color. Initially it was extremely annoying and depressing, but eventually I got used to the change just as one gets used to a scratch on an eyeglasses lens. The next few months were spent obsessively checking my vision by covering one eye and comparing them to each other. I was optimistic the damaged optic nerve would miraculously regenerate, but that proved to be a forlorn hope.

As for my definitive diagnosis of MS, the one thing that stayed with me for the first few months was the absence of lesions on the MRI of the brain. Was it possible for someone to really have MS if an MRI showed no lesions in the brain? That false sense of hope would prove to have serious consequences later that year. Over the next few months, I became proactive about finding some answers for optic neuritis, so I began looking at all the latest newsletter cures and even went for acupuncture treatments around the eye.

My only previous experience with acupuncture was a positive one that took place in 1996 in Tokyo, Japan. On the 1996 Philadelphia Orchestra tour of Asia, we performed in Seoul Korea, and the fitness center in our hotel was equipped with a state-of-the-art inversion machine. This contraption locked both ankles in a tight grip and hung one upside down like Batman for a predetermined length of time. Thinking it would be a great spinal stretch, I cleverly set the timer for five full minutes. The stretch of the spine did go as planned, but when the machine let me down I had intense back pain and was unable to move. While confined to the floor of the gym I did about twenty minutes of basic yogic back exercises before I was able to stand and walk. The orchestra tour continued but the back pain remained, and moving from city to city for the rest of the tour proved to be a major challenge. When the orchestra tour moved on to Japan, I underwent acupuncture on my back that worked amazingly well, and it was only a short time before my back felt close to normal once again.

Unfortunately, the acupuncture treatment around my left eye was not as successful as the treatment for my back had been, and the five treatments for the eye turned out to be money that would have been better spent elsewhere. To this day, I remain a firm believer in acupuncture, but not for optic neuritis.

Chapter 5

The Search for the Designer Specialist

My brother-in-law Dr. Bob Hammond, PhD was the director of the Division of Extramural Activities at the National Institute of Diabetes, Digestive and Kidney Diseases of the National Institutes of Health (NIH). I sought his advice because he is extremely knowledgeable in many fields of medicine. I explained how my diagnosis of MS was not possible because it is a disease that only affects other people. He calmed me by advising not to rush into anything after seeing just one neurologist, and he stressed the importance of getting a highly qualified second opinion. After answering several of Bob's questions, it was comforting to hear him say he would speak with the top expert on MS at the NIH, Dr. McFarland.

Dr. Henry McFarland came to the NIH as deputy chief of the Neuroimmunology Branch of the National Institute of Neurological Disorders and Stroke (NINDS) where he has served as chief since 1993. In 1998 he was awarded the Dystal Prize for outstanding research in multiple sclerosis. He was obviously a highly respected scientist who possessed a great deal of knowledge and expertise in the area of MS, and I was hopeful he would help provide the misdiagnosis I was looking for.

After speaking with Dr. McFarland, Bob instructed me to make an appointment with Dr. Fred Lublin, the top neurologist at Hahnemann Hospital and widely considered one of the three top MS specialists in the United

States. Dr. McFarland said to mention his name and give his regards to Dr. Lublin.

Dr. Fred Lublin

When I contacted the office of Dr. Lublin and mentioned Dr. Henry McFarland, it seemed to roll out the red carpet as I was given an appointment in a rather timely manner. His office was at Hahnemann Hospital in Philadelphia, where I checked in at the desk and took a seat along with his other patients. I sat in the waiting area of the office and found it disturbing to see many people with obvious advanced signs of MS. My seat was next to a man who appeared to be in his twenties, but when I struck up a conversation with him I was scared. He had great difficulty speaking because MS had affected the muscles in his face and mouth, and his resulting speech was extremely slurred. My symptoms were a non-issue compared to most of the people waiting to see Dr. Lublin, and I sat there telling myself there was no way I was going to wind up like them. In just four short months, that is exactly where I would be.

After my name was called a nurse escorted me into an examination room and said Dr. Lublin would be in shortly. After closing the door behind her, I sat nervously not knowing what to expect from this esteemed neurologist. Time always seems to pass slowly when alone in an empty examination room while anxiously waiting for the doctor to bring news of the unknown. My mind raced in hyper mode, taking in everything from the diplomas and awards on the walls to the unique smell of an examination room. When Dr. Lublin finally entered the room he seemed humored by the novelty of having a Philadelphia Orchestra cellist as a patient. After some small talk he gave me a basic neurological examination which went well, but he was intrigued by the numerous scars on my toes that were left by those mysterious blood blisters two months earlier. At this point the scars looked like someone had dotted my toes with a dull purple marker. The only place I was able to find any reference to a connection between MS and blood blisters on the toes, is a short mention in Dr. Roy Swank's famous work, The MS Diet Book.

Dr. Lublin was fixated on the scars on my toes and after a moment of silence he said the words that were music to my ears: "I have serious reservations that this is MS." At that moment he paused the examination and made a phone call to his friend Dr. Ralph DeHoratius, a well-known rheumatologist in Philadelphia. Dr. Lublin explained my situation and asked if I could get an appointment right away, but Dr. DeHoratius was booked solid and did not have an available appointment for four weeks. With the phone on his shoulder, Dr. Lublin relayed this news to me, and without hesitation I told him an earlier appointment would be rewarded with two complimentary tickets to the Philadelphia Orchestra at the Academy of Music, along with a personal backstage tour. I often wondered if I had said something that got his attention because his secretary miraculously found me an appointment that very week.

Dr. Ralph DeHoratius

Several days later when I saw Dr. DeHoratius, he gave me a basic examination and expressed an even greater interest in the scars on my toes from those previous hematomas. After a minute of reflection with his chin between his thumb and forefinger he voiced a suspicion it was vasculitis. I had never heard of vasculitis, but whatever it was, it had to be better than MS. Dr. DeHoratius proceeded with a thorough series of tests that included x-rays, blood tests and even a bone scan.

Over the next few days I was tested for everything from Lupus to mercury poisoning, along with toxicity from other heavy metals. Every one of the tests Dr. DeHoratius ordered came back negative, so rheumatoid disorders were ruled out. By the process of elimination he said it now had to be a case of MS. Shaking my head, I expressed disappointment by saying "I had hoped it was vasculitis." With a sudden look of seriousness he closed the examination room door and quietly explained, "Look, I recently lost six patients to vasculitis. Believe me when I say, it is not pretty. You are far better off with a mild case of MS than vasculitis." Feeling the blood drain from my face I breathed a sigh of relief, feeling grateful for not having been granted my wish. I later found out that vasculitis is a serious inflammation of the blood vessels. However, this was April 1999, and the next four months would prove beyond a doubt I had anything but a mild case of MS.

After ruling out all rheumatoid disorders and saying it was a mild case of MS, he sent me back to Dr. Lublin for further testing. Several days later when I saw Dr. Lublin he still had reservations about a positive diagnosis of MS because of those blood blisters on the toes. Hanging on to his doubts, I tenaciously tried to pin him down to say it was not MS. Dr. Lublin then committed to officially placing me in the "high probability category for MS," and he advised starting interferon injections. He also gave some general MS ground rules such as not exercising the muscles to the point of fatigue and avoiding cardiovascular exercise to the point of sweating.

Dr. Joan Oshinsky

At the next visit with Dr. Lublin, Dr. Joan Oshinsky, a neurologist who worked with Dr. Lublin, saw me. I knew nothing about Dr. Oshinsky, but she immediately gave the impression she was an extremely skilled neurologist. After administering the basic neurological exam she felt around at the back of my neck and said, "I think your troubles are coming from your neck." I sat there wondering how anyone could possibly know that when there had been no MRIs of my neck or spine. Since I already had MRIs of the brain, Dr. Oshinsky went with her instincts and ordered MRIs of the neck and spine.

The next time I saw Dr. Lublin, he put the MRIs of my neck and spine on the backlit screen and he pointed out three small lesions on the MRI in the neck. Dr. Lublin discussed the three lesions in the cervical spinal cord (neck area) and said he was now certain it was MS. In my continuing quest for a misdiagnosis, I pressed him about the "atypical" symptoms of those blood blisters on my toes, but he said the three small lesions in the neck were not to be argued with. The combination of numbness in one leg, vision loss in one eye and three spinal cord lesions, were a definitive diagnosis of MS. At this point Dr. Lublin said it was important to immediately begin intramuscular injections of Avonex®, which I had been advised to start by Dr. Sergott two months earlier. Not wanting to begin this drug, I asked Dr. Lublin about the risks involved if MS turned out to be a misdiagnosis. He stressed the urgency in beginning this treatment, and said there was absolutely no downside to taking the drug. Since the advice to begin the injections had come from two top MS specialists, there was little choice in the matter.

Even though I was disappointed about Dr. Lublin's definitive diagnosis, I was totally amazed that Dr. Oshinsky could possibly have found the origin of my problems from only a basic neurological exam and just feeling around at the back of my neck. Such uncanny insight strongly suggests she is a neurologist with a sixth sense of intuition.

Chapter 6

The Intramuscular Injections of Avonex®

For several years there were primarily only three drugs to treat MS, and they are known as the A-B-C drugs. Avonex®, Betaseron® and Copaxone® are all self-administered injections. The FDA approved Betaseron® in 1994, and Avonex® and Copaxone® gained FDA approval in 1996. Although other drugs have since become available, these A-B-C drugs remain commonly used to treat MS.

Avonex® is a once-a-week, self-administered intramuscular injection that is not for the faint of heart. After receiving the necessary insurance approval for the drug, a nurse came to my home to teach the intricacies of mixing the refrigerated tablet with the small bottle of saline solution before injecting it. I had to draw a measured amount of saline solution into a syringe then inject it into the tiny bottle containing the tablet. Once the tablet dissolves the mixture is drawn back into the syringe then injected deep into the muscle of the upper leg. Most people associate an injection with a much smaller and thinner needle used for subcutaneous injections (under the skin). The Avonex® intramuscular injection requires a thicker 1.25-inch needle for the needed depth into the muscle. Psychologically it was something I never quite got used to. Some nights it went smoothly but there were other nights it took almost one hour to actually get the needle into my leg.

The fear of inserting a big needle into my leg was difficult to overcome, but that was actually the easiest step with this drug. Avonex® is taken at night because the next day one is often incapacitated by the side effects. To counter the side effects, I took two ibuprofen tablets before the injection and two more tablets the next morning. I scheduled my injections on Sunday nights before bedtime because Monday was generally the orchestra's free day. The first few months on Avonex® were miserable because that next day reliably greeted me with a fever, muscle aches and intense headaches that were sheer agony. In addition, the drug temporarily inflamed both optic nerves, which further added to my vision woes.

All this time, I had done my best to keep my diagnosis of MS as quiet as possible, but word had managed to spread within the orchestra. When classical musicians hear MS, they immediately think of Jacqueline du Pré who had one of the very worst forms of the disease. When members of the orchestra asked how I was doing, I told them it was a clear misdiagnosis and what I had was unexplained. In March of 1999 Dr. Edward Viner, the orchestra's doctor and head of medicine at Cooper Hospital in Camden, NJ, saw me backstage and beat me to the punch by telling me he had already heard the news. It was difficult to believe word had traveled so quickly, but for a musician and especially a cellist to have MS, it qualified as a serious topic for water cooler conversation. Dr. Viner then asked if I would be going on the orchestra's upcoming three-week tour of Asia in May. What was surprising about his question was that he had asked with the assumption I would not be going. I was tempted to rant and rave how nothing was going to stop me, but this was backstage during intermission of an orchestra concert. Hence, I just told him that my presence on the tour was a definite.

Being on Avonex® while on the tour presented unique challenges because this medication needs to be refrigerated at all times. The drug comes in tablet form in individual small bottles and only three were needed for the entire tour. Throughout that tour I traveled with a small lunch sized insulated bag, complete with a reusable ice pack, and the airlines helped out by providing dry ice for the long flights. The Avonex® was kept refrigerated in the mini bar in each hotel room. I developed a ritual of removing the contents of the mini bar, placing everything in formation up on top. Then before checking out, I placed everything back in the same order to avoid getting charged for anything at hotel mini bar prices.

The injections while on tour required advance planning because the side effects negated the possibility of playing concerts or even traveling the next day. Luckily, the orchestra has one free day each week while on tour, so the injections went like clockwork. I had anticipated difficulty going through airport security with the big needles, but this was two and a half years before 9/11 so it was never any trouble. The first injection on the 1999 tour was particularly problematic because I had forgotten to bring the ibuprofen for the ensuing daylong flu and headache. I tried toughing out that day after my first tour injection with no ibuprofen, but it was unbearable. Not only was the headache excruciating, but the accompanying fever by the manufactured flu made things even worse. Dr. Viner who traveled with us as the orchestra's official overseas doctor, was a godsend as he helped me out for the remainder of the tour by keeping me well supplied with both Advil® and naproxen for the inflammation.

Despite the difficulties of that first tour with MS, not giving in to the disease and staying on schedule every day was a big boost of confidence. People think going on a Philadelphia Orchestra tour must be exciting and glamorous, but it is hard work considering the long flights, the jetlag, and arriving at the hotels only to find the rooms are not ready. On most days, the orchestra will fly or bus to a new city, check into the hotel around early afternoon, get dinner, play a concert, then head back to the hotel. The next day is usually a repeat of the previous day. On the tour, I never missed a rehearsal or a concert, and when I felt my worst, I bit the bullet and kept going. During this time, I was trying to convince myself I had been misdiagnosed and whatever it was that I had was mimicking the symptoms of MS.

Chapter 7

The Calm before the Storm

All went well for the next few months and there were no more symptoms from the MS, or whatever the unexplained illness was. The disease had been in remission for the five months since February, so I resumed exercising and biking with a vengeance. With each passing symptom-free day, I became further convinced MS was a misdiagnosis. I kept telling myself this was a mysterious illness whose time was short-lived, and I would never hear from it again.

Every summer since 1987 I took advantage of the Philadelphia Orchestra's optional three weeks of unpaid leave, which enabled me to teach at the Hartwick Summer Music Festival in Oneonta, NY. This beautiful place in the Catskill Mountains of upstate New York State is a cyclist's dream, so each summer I brought along both my mountain and road bikes. The summer of 1999 was different because I was on a mission to prove that MS was a misdiagnosis once and for all. To hammer the final nail in the coffin of this disease, I joined the Hartwick Summer Festival faculty group that embarked on daily 6:00 am thirty-mile cycling rides in the hills prior to the start of each day. The weather was rough that summer as the July heat and humidity were unforgiving, so the strenuous long distance hilly rides in those conditions were questionable for even a person in perfect health. For someone diagnosed with MS only five months earlier, it was dumb and downright suicidal.

The Storm

After several weeks of rigorously working out in the heat and humidity, I was abruptly rewarded with the start of my third MS attack, it was the perfect storm. Three times is the charm, and MS definitely saved the best for its third calling. This one began with the now familiar optic neuritis, but this time it targeted my right eye. The day it began, I was scheduled to play an afternoon string quartet concert for the Summer Festival. I unwisely decided not to cancel the performance.

Playing in the quartet that afternoon was an utterly miserable experience. The quartet members were Erez Ofer, the brilliant violinist and former Concertmaster of the Philadelphia Orchestra, Craig Mumm, the Associate Principal Violist of the Metropolitan Opera Orchestra, and his wife MaryAnn Mumm, who is a terrific violinist in her own right. I had been looking forward to the concert because we were playing one of the quartets by Johannes Brahms. Even though we had ample rehearsal time, my only thought during the performance was this latest loss of peripheral vision in my right eye. My left eye was still an issue because of the permanent peripheral vision and color loss, but MS had now placed my right eye in its crosshairs. Performing in a string quartet is unforgiving compared to performing in a symphony orchestra. In an orchestra, a cellist has the luxury of being assisted by nine other cellists who are playing the same part. In a string quartet, the sole cellist is expected to provide the foundation for the group, as both bass and rhythm sections. The quartet depends on the cello for everything from pitch and dynamics to depth.

During the performance of the Brahms quartet, I somehow managed to stay with the group, but I was on the defensive and there was no leading on my part. The concert took place on a hot July afternoon, in a hall with no air conditioning. While playing, my only concern was to get to the end of the last movement. Under normal circumstances, I would have been lost in the magic of Brahms. Instead, I was gripped by fear and anxiety. What was going to happen to the vision in my right eye? Would it end up worse than my left eye and would it also be permanent? How far was MS going to have its way with me unchecked?

In retrospect, playing that concert was a reckless move. I should have immediately headed home to begin intravenous steroids. This latest MS attack was particularly scary because the second attack that took place five months earlier, had gained considerably in strength over the first one. There was no way of knowing at the time, but this third attack would come in two waves, and the second wave would be tidal compared to this first one.

In a state of fright, I headed home for my second dose of intravenous steroids in five months. The routine of the steroid drip was now familiar, so it was somewhat easier this time around. Looking back with the knowledge that I gained later, drinking massive quantities of water is something I should have done in conjunction with the steroid drip. During this three-day cycle of methylprednisolone, the orders were to rest quietly and to avoid any physical activity. This proved to be a downer as the summers in Oneonta were always a great time with the bike and the cello. While this immediate intravenous steroid treatment seemed to stabilize the situation with my right eye, the respite only served to lull me into a state of complacency.

Several days after things settled down, I was hit with what seemed to be a stomach bug, and I began vomiting. Normally a stomach bug lasts only a day, but this one was proving tenacious as it kept progressing with no signs of letting up. I was unable to keep down any food or water for several days and I was constantly vomiting. My mother had come down from New York to take care of me for a few days, and I kept telling her not to call a doctor because I believed it was just a stomach bug that would soon pass. Good friends of mine, Hirono Oka, a Philadelphia Orchestra violinist, and her husband Wilbur Walmsley, heard I was pretty sick. Luckily, they stopped over for a visit. Wilbur took one look at me and immediately got on the phone with my brother-in-law Dr. Bob Hammond who was with NIH, and described my condition to him. Bob said I was showing signs of severe dehydration, and I should get to a hospital immediately. This was sound advice because I was in no physical or emotional condition to make any decisions about my health. One of my regrets in life is never having adequately expressed my gratitude to Wilbur before he passed away at an early age from lung cancer. His decision to call my brother-in-law averted what would have been a far more serious situation with lasting consequences.

While all this was going on, my colleague and cellist from the orchestra Derek Barnes and his wife Meichen, stopped by to see how I was doing. As the ambulance pulled up, Derek practically carried me outside for my ride to the hospital as I tried not to vomit on him. As soon as I got to the emergency room, they immediately inserted a catheter into my arm to replenish my dangerously low body fluids intravenously. The next four days spent in the hospital were horrible as I was now unable to see much with either eye, and the vomiting was continuing unabated. After repeated requests for something to stop the vomiting, my wish was finally granted on the second day. I took some anti-motion sickness medication that worked magic and stopped the vomiting. On my third day in the hospital, after twenty-four hours of not vomiting and seven days without food, the doctor recommended trying to eat something.

"Every fool can fast, but only a wise man can break a fast."

- George Bernard Shaw

I will never forget the first food the hospital brought me after not eating for one week – a greasy cheeseburger and French fries. It was placed on the tray over my bed and I was in a state of disbelief. There was not the slightest temptation to indulge in such a meal, and I had no doubt the vomiting would have returned with a vengeance. This is a questionable meal even for a healthy person, but in my physical state it would have been sheer insanity. George Bernard Shaw would certainly have had some new witticism for whomever it was that took the liberty of ordering that first meal after my fast.

Luckily, I was able to get a macrobiotic lunch delivered from Center Foods in Philadelphia, a place that unfortunately no longer exists. Admittedly, part of my draw to this place was the unofficial dress code: none of the female employees wore bras. This small family run place was one of the most serious health food stores and cafes I had ever been to, and seeing it close several years later was a truly sad day in my life.

Keeping that first meal down was a milestone, so I was discharged from the hospital after four days. It felt great to be home and out of the hospital because they were doing little other than giving me IV fluids and checking vital signs several times each day. The hospital seemed delighted to have me as a guest because my condition required little attention from the doctors, nurses and staff. Room and board were covered by my health insurance provider, and I was not even eating the food. In comparison to the other patients at the hospital, I certainly qualified as a cheap date.

To this day, missing the Philadelphia Orchestra's 1999 Saratoga Performing Arts Center summer festival in Saratoga Springs, NY still emotionally haunts me. I have been to many wonderful places on the planet, but Saratoga is definitely one of my favorites. My first time in Saratoga was in the summer of 1975, when I attended the School of Orchestral Studies program for high school students. That experience transformed my life from a kid with little direction, to one of a highly self-motivated cellist. It was here I first took private lessons from the Philadelphia Orchestra's principal cellist William Stokking, and he was the incredibly passionate and motivating teacher I needed. This was my first opportunity to study cello with someone at such a high professional level, and this is only one of my many magical memories from Saratoga. In my thirty years with the Philadelphia Orchestra, I never missed a tour, and I only missed one summer in Saratoga, which was August 1999 when I was hospitalized.

Dr. Fred Lublin was still my neurologist during the time I was hospitalized, but I had not seen him in four months. My last visit with him was back in April when he confirmed it was MS and started me on Avonex®. There was a phone in the hospital room and despite three days of repeated calls to his office, I was unable to reach him. One can imagine the level of frustration of being in that situation and not being able to reach their neurologist. Unbeknownst to me at the time, Hahnemann Hospital was experiencing dire financial difficulties and they were in the process of closing their Department of Neurology. To make matters worse Dr. Lublin had accepted a position with a hospital in Manhattan and he was in the process of relocating to New York City. When he finally returned my call he was calm about my situation, but I was in a complete state of panic. What a neurologist regularly sees as a common occurrence with MS is a very different picture than what the patient sees. I had hoped Dr. Lublin would take an active role giving direction, by speaking with my hospital neurologist or having me transferred to Hahnemann; but none of this was meant to happen. He was not overly concerned about a "flare up," and said to come see him when I got out of the hospital.

At this point I felt the need for a neurologist who would be more readily accessible, so I called Dr. Edward Viner, the Philadelphia Orchestra's overseas touring doctor, and he set up an appointment with Dr. Clyde Markowitz of the Hospital of the University of Pennsylvania (HUP) in Philadelphia. At the time, Dr. Viner was the Director of Medicine at Cooper Hospital in Camden, NJ, so he was able to get me in to see Dr. Markowitz without delay. Dr. Viner said Dr. Markowitz was a top-notch neurologist and felt I would do well with him. That timely appointment was badly needed both physically and psychologically. I had just been released from the hospital and had no idea where to turn next. This was my absolute lowest point in terms of debilitation. The use of my hands was at a near total loss, and my vision was limited to seeing only silhouettes. The nausea and vomiting were somewhat under control by the anti-motion sickness medication I was given at the hospital, but they were kept at bay only by a hair. I was able to walk, but with great difficulty and only for very short distances. Because the optic neuritis was riding the wave, the impaired vision even made shaving a challenge. It was impossible to see individual hairs on my face and because my hands had no feeling, there was no way to tell if I was clean-shaven. Urinating and defecating had become an ordeal because there was almost no sensation of when the processes began and when they ended. Even finishing the paperwork after a bowel movement was extremely difficult, and it was accomplished with a good amount of guesswork.

Frustration with my Neurologist

I know several people with MS who became extremely frustrated with their neurologist, and I can fully understand because I was one of them. I saw five different neurologists during my first eight months with MS, and I ended up staying with the fifth one. Throughout our lives, we see doctors for various ailments and illnesses. We expect the doctor to diagnose, prescribe the appropriate medication, surgery or physical therapy, then we get better. Unfortunately things are not that simple when it comes to neurological disorders, and MS is particularly good at driving people to an extreme degree of frustration.

It took two full months after my initial symptoms before I received my first diagnosis of MS. In the first four months after the first signs of the disease, there were visits to a family doctor, an orthopedic surgeon, a neurosurgeon and two neurologists. I did not believe the initial diagnosis because the MRI of the brain was clear of lesions, but the reality was that I was not willing to believe it. Two months later, my second neurologist found three small lesions in the spinal cord and said it was definitely MS. I was still reluctant to accept it and I successfully implored him to place me in the high probability category for the disease. It took another six months, a vicious attack and lesions in the MRIs of my brain that resembled streetlights to convince me it actually was MS. It is easy to become frustrated and blame a neurologist, but how can one expect a neurologist to treat a patient who refuses to accept the diagnosis? MS is a neurological disorder that affects each person differently and there is no way of predicting how each patient will fare. In many cases, the neurologist is the one who winds up taking the blame.

Chapter 8

My First Visit with Dr. Clyde Markowitz

I first saw Dr. Clyde Markowitz on August 16, 1999, five days after being released from a four-day hospital stay for dehydration. The thirty-five-minute car ride to the Hospital of the University of Pennsylvania for this initial visit was miserable. I was in the front passenger seat of the car and the ride triggered a serious and unprepared reversal of fortune. The anti-motion sickness medication I was given at the hospital succeeded in keeping the vomiting at bay, but this car ride through the city of Philadelphia in August was too much to bear. Since my car was not equipped with an air sickness bag, I poked my head out the window and proceeded to decorate the side of the car with a creative psychedelic design.

As I stumbled into the lobby of HUP, the guard and the people at the front desk saw me struggling and quickly determined a wheelchair would be in order. They brought one out, sat me down and directed me to the Department of Neurology. Sitting in the waiting area of HUP's department of Neurology brought back memories of my first visit to Dr. Lublin's office back in April. Several of Dr. Markowitz's patients in the room were dealing with seriously advanced cases of MS that were on par with Dr. Lublin's patients. Four months earlier, I sat in the waiting area of Dr. Lublin's office certain my case was a misdiagnosis, and knowing I would never have to deal with anything close to what his patients were dealing with. How ironic it was that I was now the one sitting in a wheelchair, almost blind and barely able to use my hands.

While sitting there waiting to see Dr. Markowitz, I was immersed in self-pity and wondering why all this was happening to me. Then a nurse interrupted my misery to wheel me into one of the examination rooms. Once there I sat in the silent room feeling like an injured mouse that was being toyed with by a cat just before the fatal bite. I just could not believe what MS had accomplished with such brutality and efficiency in eight short months.

Dr. Markowitz then entered the room, introduced himself, and sat down to read my chart while the clock slowly ticked away. After several minutes he looked up and said with a smile, "I understand you are a concert cellist." After my recent attempt to play Bach on the cello, there were serious doubts if any truth existed in his words, but I was hopeful he would somehow work a miracle and give me my life back. This was the fifth neurologist I had seen in six months and maybe he was the magician who would pull a rabbit out of his hat and stop this ruthless disease from destroying my body and my life any further.

Dr. Markowitz then proceeded with a series of basic neurological tests and the results were not good. My eyes and hands were the main targets of this attack and his tests confirmed what I already knew. One notable test failure was when I closed my eyes and was unable to tell if he was bending my toes and fingers up or down. The vision with my eyes open was not much better than with them closed because the optic nerves were so inflamed it was a struggle to see anything. When he instructed me to walk across the room I managed with great difficulty, but when he said to stand still with eyes closed I lost my balance and stumbled. Realizing the seriousness of the situation, Dr. Markowitz took a very active role and immediately ordered a complete set of MRIs and blood work to see where things stood.

The most disturbing results of all the tests were the images of the brain and spinal cord. He said my MRIs showed "numerous active lesions in the brain and spinal cord" and my brain was "all lit up." The numerous lesions and my horrendous physical condition alarmed Dr. Markowitz to the point he put me on a ten-day course of intravenous steroids. Back in February and July of 1999, I had been on three-day doses, but 1,000 milligrams of intravenous steroids every day for ten days? It seemed radical at the time, but Dr. Markowitz was right on target as my body responded very well to that seemingly insane dose of steroids, and it succeeded in immediately stopping my vicious third attack dead in its tracks.

It should be noted that Dr. Markowitz is a truly excellent neurologist in every respect. From the beginning, he displayed superior people-person skills, which are invaluable to someone who is fragile and panicked. He never treated me like a nuisance and the best part was his personal return of every one of my phone calls in a timely manner. On one occasion, he returned one of my calls during his lunch break and I could hear him eating throughout the conversation. When a neurologist calls his patients during his lunch hour, it is a testament to a dedicated and passionate health professional who cares for his patients. During the office visits, he listened to my ideas that were good and bad, and he did so with an open mind and without prejudice. Neurologists as a group may have a "diagnose and adios" reputation, but this does not apply to Dr. Markowitz because he took a personal interest in my case even when it looked hopeless. Any neurologist would find it easy to take a special interest in my case now, but Dr. Markowitz gets credit for the hard part.

Chapter 9

PEDs - Performance Enhanced Dreams

Perhaps some of today's professional athletes would be envious of a potent ten-day dose of intravenous steroids, but in my case, it was a different kind of steroid and there were no performance-enhancing benefits. It was a necessary evil and it was my only chance of arresting the cruel effects of that third attack. I spent that extended period on steroids lying in bed with no music, television or entertainment of any kind. The anxiety of having everything stolen rendered it impossible to do things that would normally help pass the hours. The time elapsed in slow motion and I was in a zone somewhere between life and death, similar to Count Dracula spending his days hidden from the light.

The ten-day, steroid-induced, semi-vegetative prison, felt like I was shackled and in solitary confinement. During that time, there was one continuous burning desire – to get back on the bike. Even more than playing the cello again, I wanted to move fast on two wheels and feel the wind on my face. While lying in bed I yearned to relive that first moment when I learned to balance on two wheels of a bicycle. Riding a bike without training wheels is a child's first taste of freedom in the world, and I was desperate to feel that same freedom once again. After following Lance Armstrong's Tour de France victories and seeing what getting back on the bike did for him, I was convinced that it would be a major help both physically and psychologically.

There was no shortage of bad dreams to keep me company during the ten days on intravenous steroids. The single worst memory during that time was a nightmare that occurred in the middle of the day, toward the end of the ten days. Everything about the dream was so real, and it left me unsettled with a dream hangover for quite some time. It took place at my own viewing in a funeral home. I was lying in an open casket with my eyes closed and both arms folded across my chest. In classic dream form, I was able to view everything from some non-specific vantage point. Many mourners were present at my viewing and I did not recognize a single person. The women who were present at my service were dressed in black and they were loudly crying behind their veils. I awoke from the dream screaming and the house was eerily quiet. The nightmare seemed more real than the present. The filtered sunlight entering the bedroom was the same as it was in the funeral home. At first, I thought death had come for me and this was the afterlife, but after a moment, I realized it was only a dream.

Considering the massive dose of steroids I was on, the side effects were minimal and the only major issue aside from the dreams was an infected elbow as the result of immunosuppressant complications. After the intravenous steroids were finished and while tapering down with the oral prednisone, my right elbow became painfully swollen and turned an angry red color. It was particularly disturbing because there had been no mishap or injury to cause such an infection. At the first sign of this latest trouble, I called Dr. Markowitz and he saw me that very day. He immediately prescribed some heavy antibiotics that successfully cleared up the bizarre and ugly infection.

Chapter 10

The Fight Begins

My August 1999 Visit with Dr. Robert Sergott

I first saw Dr. Sergott at Wills Eye Hospital in February 1999. Since that time, I had monitoring checkups with him on a regular basis over the next six months. He tested me for everything imaginable, including numerous blood tests for everything from Lyme disease to heavy metal toxicity. He also ordered several MRIs, a chest x-ray, a bone scan and a neurological conduction test (also known as NCV or nerve conduction velocity test). Seeing the results of each test was a relief because each one came back normal.

Dr. Sergott monitored the condition of my eyes by testing basic vision as well as visual field. When neuritis strikes the optic nerve, peripheral vision is commonly the first to go, as it was in my case. To measure my exact amount of peripheral vision loss, Dr. Sergott administered a visual field test. For anyone who has never had a visual field test, here is a quick primer. The lights in the room are turned off and the patient looks into something similar to the eyepiece of a periscope. One eye is covered with a patch while the other eye looks through the eyepiece and focuses on a central point on a video screen. The patient is given an electronic thumb clicker to hold while focusing on that central point. When tiny lights quickly flash in the periphery of that central point, the patient responds with a click of the thumb. A test score is calculated by the number of flashes that are followed by a click of the thumb.

Dr. Sergott kept track of my condition during the four months between my second and third exacerbations, and I felt lucky the results were continuously stable. During that period of time I went to Wills Eye Hospital for so many tests and with such frequency, that I joked about tipping the doorman. For quite some time the peripheral vision and color loss in my left eye were a nuisance and it felt like I would never get used to it. I was among the many who always took good vision for granted, and I now feel somewhat ungrateful for having done so. Dr. Sergott was quite helpful in calming my frustration when he advised adjusting to the new vision by comparing it to a scratch on an eyeglass lens. The scratch is initially bothersome, but after some time the scratch is no longer noticed. At first, it was extremely difficult not to dwell on the peripheral vision loss, but eventually I managed to do so and I no longer notice it. The visits with Dr. Sergott were routine because there was no change from February 1999 until July of that year.

My appointment with Dr. Sergott in August 1999 was a major mile-marker in my journey. I had recently been released from the hospital and I was in extremely poor condition. It was my absolute lowest and worst point with MS. However, this was also the point where I decided enough was enough and the gloves would now come off. I remember this visit quite well, and to say it went badly would be an understatement. I was in a horrendous physical state and my emotional state was far worse. The three MS attacks during the eight-month period all came without warning and each one was progressively stronger. At the time of this visit, walking half a block was as difficult as running a marathon because my body was seriously lacking physical strength. I informed Dr. Sergott that I had started with yet another neurologist, the latest being Dr. Markowitz at HUP. I also kept him up to date on Dr. Markowitz's putting me on 1000 mg of intravenous methylprednisolone for ten straight days. Dr. Sergott seemed shocked by such a high dose of intravenous steroids as if he had never heard of someone getting that amount for ten days, but Dr. Sergott's next two tests would clearly illustrate just how far my case of MS had progressed since the time of our last visit.

Dr. Sergott began by administering a basic vision test and the results were a total failure. I was unable to read the letters on the vision chart – even the very largest ones. He then positioned me in the chair for a visual field test by placing the thumb clicker in my hand and instructed me to click each time a light flashed. I knew the routine well but when the test commenced, I sat in the chair and focused on the screen without clicking because there were no flashing lights in the periphery. After a short time, Dr. Sergott paused the test and resumed it with my other eye, but it was no better. I sat there frozen once again without a single click. After prematurely stopping the visual field test, Dr. Sergott wheeled his chair over to his desk with his back to me and proceeded to write on my chart for what seemed like an eternity. Then he turned and said something I will never forget, "I will write you a note for permanent disability."

Time suddenly stopped. In slow motion my nonexistent future began playing out on a screen before me. Unable to use my hands or eyes I sat there shell shocked, as if I had just been stabbed through the heart with a knife. For good measure, the stab with this knife was followed up with a twist. My situation had gone from a state of denial where I feared my colleagues in the orchestra would learn I had MS, to the point where I would be on permanent disability and no longer able to play the cello. My surroundings suddenly changed to a courtroom in a foreign country where a judge just read my death sentence. There would be no phone call to a lawyer, no continuance, and no stay of execution granted by this court. Once again I thought of the brilliant cellist Jacqueline du Pré, who died of complications from the disease at the age of forty-two. Dr. Sergott's words "I will write you a note for permanent disability," were being interpreted differently by my brain: "Your life is over. You have gone from a person who supported society, to one whom society will support. Your life will now be the waiting room before the cemetery." I was Ebenezer Scrooge, Dr. Sergott was the ghost of Christmas future, and he had just shown me my grave.

Suddenly things began moving in real time as I was hit with a startling surge of energy. This was not going to happen and there was no way I was going down that road. Refusing to accept Dr. Sergott's prognosis, I snapped at him in a moment of anger, "You can take that note and use it as a suppository because I'm going back to work in six weeks when the orchestra's season starts." He looked at me in disbelief, apparently offended by such a rude and disrespectful patient. He came right back with a sharp retort:

"How are you going to do that?"

"Well, I am going back to work!" I said.

Now I radiated only a mix of anger and tears and Dr. Sergott seeing I was obviously upset, tried to calm me by saying the following words that would change the equation, "I have to tell you, I've seen people in your position a year from now and they're still in a wheelchair, and I've seen people in your position a year from now and you wouldn't know anything is wrong with them." My response was instant. "Well I'm going to be one of those people a year from now, and you won't know anything is wrong with me."

I would spend the next few years reflecting on Dr. Sergott's words because he unknowingly left me a choice. How I would wind up in one year would not be left to fate or happenstance. Dr. Sergott gave me the chance to take the initiative and determine my outcome. Those words were invaluable and I credit him for being one of the key people who helped me get my life back. He also recommended getting on the common antidepressant Prozac, and explained it would be unnatural for someone with such a severe case of MS to not go into a serious depression. He took out his prescription pad and wrote me a script for Prozac which I placed in my pocket but never filled. In retrospect, I wish he had written the letter for permanent disability, because it would now be in a frame and proudly displayed on my wall.

Because I was dead serious about going back to work and resuming a normal life, Dr. Sergott stressed the importance of taking good care of myself. "You have to be serious about this. If at any point you are not feeling well, it is important to take two or three days off and rest." But I did exactly the opposite. Over the next few years and particularly on the days I felt the worst, I refused to let it affect me one bit. I forced myself to get moving each day to proceed with a full day of work. In fact, there were few days during the first year of my recovery when I felt even remotely close to well.

In addition to feeling horrible most of the time, I spent one day each week wrestling with the side effects of Avonex®. The day after every injection felt like a case of the flu so bad that my hair hurt. Despite all the challenges, I made up my mind that nothing was going to stop me from now on – *nothing!* I finally forced myself to accept the diagnosis but I would never accept the prognosis. This so-called "incurable illness" was finally going to meet its match!

As it turned out, not taking the antidepressant helped keep my mind sharp and tuned in to those intricate signals the body sends to the brain. A major downside to declining the antidepressant was the heavy toll that was taken on the relationship with my children. It was impossible to accept what had happened to my body and life, and I became an extremely angry and frustrated person. A devastating illness can affect a family in many ways. It can strengthen bonds between loved ones just as easily as it can tear them apart. After I was released from the hospital, during what was already turning out to be the absolute worst time in my life in the first place, I had one of the worst fights imaginable with my former wife. She stormed out of the house, and at that moment I knew my only chance of survival was to be on my own. It was hard to imagine what impact the diagnosis was having on the people around me, as I was struggling to come to terms with it myself. Six months after the misery of that fight, I passed by a house which was located one block away from where we lived and there was a "for rent" sign on the lawn. I knew the owners of the house because their daughter babysat my kids several years before. I was very close with both of my children and this seemed like the perfect solution. I imagined that they could come and go as they pleased and there would be no need for them to be driven back and forth from house to house. The next day I signed a one-year lease on my new place. I had envisioned the new living arrangement as a perfect solution for a broken home with children, but I was naive. The situation had a negative impact on both children because the only life they knew had been torn apart. At the time my daughter was 12, my son was 10 and they were both too young to fully understand the desperateness of my situation. The insidiousness of MS had my dream life, my "happily ever after" collapsing from underneath me in every possible way.

Most of the time, I managed to keep my anger and frustration bottled up, but admittedly there were times I took it out on my children by becoming unreasonable and raising my voice. The one thing I will always be grateful for is never having repeated my father's mistake of beating his children. This is definitely one of those instances where one wishes life had that elusive rewind button. If it did I would go back and spend time explaining to my children the challenges and extreme difficulties of fighting MS. I have a feeling my son Ryan, who became a professional Mixed Martial Arts (MMA) fighter, must have some understanding of what I went through considering what he does for a living. Life can be cruel at times, particularly when it wields a double-edged sword.

Accept the Diagnosis - Reject the Prognosis

I made the decision to refuse to accept a prognosis of permanent disability under duress during an emotional burst of anger. It is a decision that saved my life. I know in my heart if the choice had been disability or even an extended period of sick leave, it would have been the end. Throughout life, we face major decisions that affect us for the rest of our lives. Some situations give us time to think and plan before we commit, and other situations demand an immediate answer. In many instances if one guesses right they are a genius, and if one guesses wrong they are a loser.

MS was now part of me. There could be no more denying it or lying about it to others. More importantly, there would be no more lying to myself. MS may have had its way by winning the first three battles, but it would now lose the war. Until this point it had a perfect 3-for-3 record against me. Now, I would not sit around waiting for a grand slam fourth attack. I was totally unprepared and taken by surprise during the first three battles, but from now on, I would take the initiative and MS would be placed on the defensive. Anything and everything in my life would now be devoted to being armed to the teeth with superior weapons and firepower. This opponent would blink first and wave the white flag.

Chapter 11

Spinal Tap

Dr. Markowitz is a highly respected neurologist because he is thorough and does not overlook things, but what I like most about him is his open-mindedness. Once the intravenous steroids had succeeded in arresting my third attack, Dr. Markowitz took the opportunity to work his magic. Taking advantage of a cease-fire, he began extensive testing to find out exactly what was going on. In addition to the long list of standard tests for someone in my condition, he wanted to see what was in my spinal fluid so he prescribed a spinal tap. When I asked when and where the procedure would be performed, I was surprised when he said he would do it himself right then and there in the office. Having never had a spinal tap, I was somewhat shy of the concept of having a needle inserted into my spine to withdraw fluid. After forewarning of an ensuing headache Dr. Markowitz gave the instructions to pull up my shirt, bend over and sit motionless for the insertion of the needle and filling of the syringe. I was mentally prepared for some intense pain from the procedure, but surprisingly his skilled and steady hands produced almost no sensation.

About 30 minutes after the procedure, I left the office with no headache. I felt lucky to have been spared the misery. However, after another 15 minutes I was anything but lucky because a headache set in, and it was not pleasant. I took a few ibuprofen tablets to ease the pain but it was not much help. This headache was different from any I had ever experienced as it had a strange and artificial feeling, one that could be described as a medically induced headache. As I waited patiently for the unnatural throbbing to subside, an unexpected swelling of the spinal cord set in and it mercilessly kept me company for the next two weeks. Those two weeks turned out to be among the most miserable and painful weeks of my life.

Swelling of the spinal cord was accompanied by an excruciating and constant headache from hell. The only respite was to lie down and not move. The headache immediately following the spinal tap was bad, but it was only a little teaser compared to this one. Keeping my head upright, for even a short period, was indescribably painful. The throbbing was just too intense. Getting up, even for a quick trip to the bathroom, was painful. It felt like I was being pounded on the head with a wooden mallet. So, I spent the next two weeks alternating between the couch and the bed, with only fast trips to the bathroom to break up the monotony. It seemed like the longest two weeks I can remember. The time passed in agonizingly slow motion and it seemed it would never end. It is a commonly known fact that the human brain has no memory for pain, but I distinctly remember the pain from that headache during those two miserable weeks.

Moral of the story: Next time a doctor tells me to get a spinal tap, I'll go see the cult classic movie *This is Spinal Tap* instead!

Chapter 12

Back on the Bike for the First Time

After the hospital stay and the ten days on intravenous steroids had concluded, it was time to fulfill that burning desire to get back on the bike. The one obstacle I faced with a bike ride was the current state of my central nervous system, which gave serious doubts to the possibility of balancing on two wheels. Even if balancing on a bicycle was still possible, a bigger issue would be my eyesight. My extremely limited vision and impaired peripheral vision made it difficult to differentiate between moving and parked cars. I was able to see the shapes of cars but my limited depth perception made it hard to tell if an object was sitting still or in motion. Many years earlier, I spent a good deal of time teaching my children Amanda and Ryan how to ride a bike, but now it was their turn to help me relearn the skill. In preparation for the first ride, I lowered the seat to its minimum height. For safety, there would be no using the clip-in pedals I had grown accustomed to. In addition to a helmet, I wore heavy padded gloves as a precautionary measure against any unexpected rendezvous with the pavement. The game plan was for Amanda and Ryan to be my guides by starting out in front. I would follow their silhouettes and shout for help if I fell. I pushed off on the mountain bike, began pedaling and to my surprise I was able to balance on the bike. It was a great feeling that was reminiscent of my euphoric victory ride as a child when I successfully balanced on two wheels for the first time. That first bike ride after my hospital stay lasted only a few blocks, but the die was cast. The skill of balancing on two wheels had not been lost, and from this point, I would gradually begin rebuilding my strength and endurance. The successful bike ride was a needed boost of confidence as it shined a glimmer of promising light at the end of a long dark tunnel. I could relate to what Orville Wright must have felt after his historic 12-second, 120-foot flight. I did not change the future of the world in a way Orville and Wilbur Wright did, but I changed my own future. The Wright brothers made history by being the first to fly, but my first bicycle ride after the third MS attack was one step better – it was longer than 12 seconds and farther than 120 feet.

The Walk to Middle School

Despite the triumph of being in the saddle again, I was still facing major challenges. In early September 1999, just three weeks after getting out of the hospital, my daughter Amanda started middle school in Cherry Hill, NJ, which was exactly one-half mile from where we lived. At this point walking was incredibly difficult but I made up my mind to walk her to school whenever possible. My 10-day intravenous steroid treatment had concluded and it was now the middle of my six-week tapering-down period with oral prednisone. To counter the effects of the massive levels of steroids in my system I began drinking more water than I previously did. The very first round-trip walk to school was disastrous because there had been no planning for incontinence issues. With my body in such a raw and fragile state, the walk was exhausting. In retrospect, I should have visited the bathroom at the school. As it turned out, the last tenth of a mile of that walk home proved to be a losing battle. I tried in vain to hold my bladder, but one block from home I wet myself and it was an absolutely miserable feeling. This was no minor mishap, but a major one. To wet your pants as a child is one thing, but to wet your pants at the age of forty is a different story.

Losing control of my bladder was a physical and psychological setback, and my goal of re-establishing my position with the orchestra in two weeks was not looking realistic. That round-trip walk to school was just over thirty minutes and I wasn't even able to hold my bladder for such a short time. That warm experience of wetting myself did not bode well for managing the hold time before intermission of an orchestra rehearsal or a concert. Wetting my pants brought back two painful memories from childhood that I still vividly remember. One of those unpleasant experiences happened after seeing a horror movie that seemed frighteningly real at the time. The other was at the hands of my father when I was being disciplined.

Weighing My Options

August 1999 resembled the aftermath of nuclear war. Essentially, I was left without the use of my eyes or fingers, and my body felt like it was receiving a constant low voltage stream of electric current. Despite all the challenges I faced, two commitments were made to Dr. Sergott and I was determined to live up to them:

1. In just six weeks, I would rejoin the Philadelphia Orchestra for the start of the 1999-2000 season.

2. One year from now Dr. Sergott would not know there was anything wrong with me.

During the following weeks, my thoughts were consumed with achieving the goal of getting my life back, but I had no idea how this was going to be accomplished. MS is an incurable disease with an enviable track record. It seemed the best hope for most people was to get it into remission, keep it under control and learn to live with it. This was unacceptable to me so I made up my mind to do the impossible – to beat MS outright. There were several options on the table, and in retrospect it was wise to have given careful thought to each option just as a chess player analyzes possibilities. In the game of chess, a skilled player considers the consequences of each move before it is made. The highly skilled and successful chess player will think and plan further ahead than an opponent. Competing against MS is similar to chess in many ways, but the real difference is MS is not a game. If I lost this contest, the game was over – for good.

Taking time to think and plan is important not only in chess, but in all aspects of life. When dealing with a major health crisis, thought and planning can mean the difference between life and death. Since I have beaten MS, many people have contacted me asking if I would please speak to a loved one who has recently been diagnosed with the disease. I am always happy to help because my first year with the disease would have benefitted greatly by what I now know. When I attempt to contact that recently diagnosed loved one, I am not surprised when they do not want to speak to anyone about their situation – including me. I can relate to that mindset because I was there. In addition to not wanting to speak to anyone about my MS diagnosis, I was in a complete state of denial. I even lied about it to people. An MS diagnosis is truly a crisis, and that is the time when a personal advisor of sorts would be most helpful. To shed some light on that theory, one only has to look at political scandals that take the stage in the eyes of the public. It is interesting how some politicians manage to successfully weather intense political storms while others do not. The biggest political scandal I remember during my childhood was when a well-connected U.S. Senator drove his car off a bridge in Massachusetts and his passenger did not survive. Before taking any immediate action, he went home and did not report the incident until the next day. The time he took to clear his mind and body, to think and plan before saying anything, no doubt saved a political career. A more modern famous political scandal involved an inappropriate relationship between the President and a White House intern. In that case, spin-doctors were set in motion before any words were said and before any action was taken. Careful planning was initiated and another political career was spared. It is no exaggeration to say methodical thinking, planning and discipline spared my life. I may have had a reactive mindset for my first eight months with MS, but a vicious third attack and a prognosis of permanent disability changed everything. That was the point when my mindset and approach changed, and I committed to thinking and planning my way out of a major health crisis.

The following options received careful thought and consideration:

Suicide

In August of 1999, my situation was so hopeless that suicide initially seemed like the only option. How does a person realistically come to terms with an eight-month transition from a normal, healthy and successful life to one where an incurable disease has taken everything away? The thought of suicide did cross my mind, but that would have meant giving up without a fight. In addition it would have inflicted great pain and suffering on those left behind. Suicide was ruled out because I somehow felt hope even though there was no visible light at the end of the tunnel. The only possible benefit from the option of suicide would have been the seven-figure life insurance policy that would have provided for the future needs of my two children. Their financial future would have been secured but it would have been eclipsed by the trauma of such an action. It would have meant saddling both of them with associated baggage that they would carry with them for the rest of their lives.

Go on permanent disability and not return to the orchestra.

A former member of the Philadelphia Orchestra had taken this road, but in that particular case, it appeared to be only for self-serving purposes. The situation was particularly troubling because this person allegedly belittled his colleagues by saying they "didn't know how to take advantage of the system." The validity of disability in that situation was highly dubious, as there seemed to be little consideration for right and wrong. The entire orchestra was aghast by their perception of a lack of self-respect, and for this reason alone the option was off the table. The severity of my illness definitely validated permanent disability but there was not the slightest temptation to take this road. Permanent disability is a choice I could not have lived with, and in my case, it very possibly would have led to the first option of suicide. For me, permanent disability was an early resignation. If there was any possible way of regrouping and rejoining society as a productive member, I had to try it with everything I had.

Go on temporary disability and fight the MS by taking one of the A-B-C drugs.

My third attack came after I had been on the drug Avonex® for four months, and I was having doubts about the drug's efficacy in my case. It was now August 1999 and the third attack did not seem the slightest bit phased by the drug. When I was hospitalized for dehydration and motion sickness I stopped taking the Avonex®, but at my first visit with Dr. Markowitz he made it quite clear that I should resume taking it immediately. At that initial appointment with my newest neurologist, I was in no frame of mind to argue so I followed his advice and promptly resumed the injections that very day. As for the option of temporary disability or taking sick leave, a voice inside was telling me to get back to my normal way of life as soon as possible without taking any time off. This approach no doubt must have seemed radical to my doctors, but I felt there was no choice if this disease was going to be beaten. Going back to the orchestra was anything but easy but I followed through with my commitment and rejoined the group for the start of the 1999 – 2000 season. Looking back, I am convinced it was the right choice and it definitely helped get my life back.

Decline the disability and take one of the A-B-C drugs.

This did seem like an option but I had doubts about how much the Avonex® was actually helping. There had to be more than just taking one of the A-B-C drugs and waiting around with the hope things would get better. Because my mindset was more proactive than reactive, this option appeared limited. It will always be impossible to place a finger on exactly what was responsible for my complete victory over MS, but to this day I give a great deal of credit to my steadfast refusal to give in, not even for one minute.

Decline the disability, decline the A-B-C drugs and go with the homeopathic approach.

This option meant giving up one of the best treatments Western medicine offered for MS at the time. When I went to see Dr. Ronald Hoffman in New York and met with Jodi Gelfand, his physician's assistant, her advice was to "stack the deck in my favor from every possible angle." Having complete faith and trust in Jodi came naturally as she radiated genuineness and a motherly concern that is a rarity among health professionals. Jodi advised staying on the Avonex® along with all the supplements Dr. Hoffman had recommended. Avonex® is not a cure, but it does have a proven track record of slowing down the progression of MS. At this point, giving up on this drug would have been a serious gamble, with the risks far outweighing the rewards. Therefore, I eliminated this option.

Decline the disability and combine one of the A-B-C drugs with the homeopathic approach.

This was an option that I liked, but once again there were limits. I met several people with MS that followed this route, but in their cases, the MS slowly progressed. This option was also not good enough as I wanted something better and knew I could get more by adding to this option.

Decline the disability, aggressively hydrate the body, clean up the diet, take one of the A-B-C drugs, research homeopathic treatments, rebuild the body with exercise and learn mind control to make changes within the body.

With good reason, this is the one I finally settled on. This is what Jodi Gelfand meant when she said to stack the deck in my favor from every possible angle. It would take hard work and discipline, but the key word was persistence. No matter how bad things looked, I could never give up. I made the decision to not only go with this option, but also to give it everything I had. Whatever needed to be sacrificed would go. There would be no looking back. When I jumped into this option with both feet, there was absolutely no light at the end of a long dark tunnel. However, over the next few weeks and months a faint light began to emerge in the distance, and it appeared slightly brighter each day. Over the next few months, MS not only stopped progressing, but things even began showing some signs of improvement.

Chapter 13

The Research Begins

The Problem:

How does a person who is seriously debilitated with MS resume a normal life in six weeks and cure the disease?

The Solution:

There was no known solution. Going back to work in six weeks was one thing, but curing MS was considered impossible. My journey would take place in uncharted territory and much of it would be trial and error.

I had been on the intramuscular injections of Avonex® for the past four months and at that time, it was widely accepted as one of the best treatments for a person in my predicament. Other than the two-week break when I was hospitalized, I never missed the weekly injections. Despite that, they had not slowed the progression of the disease as I had hoped. The third attack was full scale and it effectively disabled much of my central nervous system, leaving parts of my body useless.

Fear of the unknown was omnipresent. There was constant anxiety of when the next attack would hit and what surprise would be up its sleeve. Prior to that third attack, I read several books written by people with MS. It seemed the common theme was to accept the disease and hope to get it into remission. This philosophy of making room in my life for MS was unacceptable because in nine short months it had been ruthless, and I had no interest in keeping this horrible disease as a permanent freeloading roommate. I wanted it out of my body and was determined to find some way of getting rid of it.

My vision was so poor that reading books was out of the question therefore the local library would be of no help. One redeeming feature turned out to be enlarging the font on my 21-inch computer screen, which finally made reading possible. This proved a lifesaver as I now began the research that would help achieve my immediate goal of going back to work in six weeks. My basic research began with everything I could find about MS. This included statistics from different countries on all different latitudes and longitudes, possible causes, holistic and folk remedies, foods to eat or avoid, and activities that would help or hurt. The internet was an outstanding tool for research because there was no censorship by special interests, and I had access to just about everything. I found a wealth of helpful online information, and to this day I wonder if my complete recovery could have been possible without modern internet access.

I had no medical knowledge and knew even less when it came to chemistry, biology and pharmacology. One thing I did know was the very best Western medicine treatments for MS offered only the hope of slowing the progression of the disease, or at best keeping it in remission. Therefore, I would have to find obvious answers that modern neurology and Western medicine had overlooked. One major advantage I had was something that I accomplished 24 years earlier: my commitment to become a serious cellist. This would later prove to be a major help in fighting the disease.

I started playing the cello in third grade at my public elementary school at the age of nine and immediately displayed a talent for the instrument. Unfortunately, my interest in the cello dissipated after a short time and I spent the next few years fighting with my mother whenever she told me to practice. Worse than not being serious about the cello, was my persistent contentiousness with my mother because I wanted to quit. To this day it is incomprehensible how or why she put up with such an ungrateful little brat. No one else in my family played an instrument. Classical music was not part of my family culture and I resented being the only child in the household who was singled out to play an instrument. Things changed in the seventh grade when I discovered the guitar and began teaching myself how to play. In the process, I rediscovered a love for music that had been dormant for several years and luckily, I focused my time and energy on the guitar. This was a more natural fit due to my familiarity with popular music and the surrounding peer pressure. I became quite serious with the guitar and practiced for several hours each day. Within two years, I was the lead guitarist in my first of several rock bands.

In August 1975 at age sixteen, things changed again when I received a letter about the School of Orchestral Studies which was a four-week program in Saratoga, NY. This caught my attention because teachers in the program were members of the Philadelphia Orchestra. This was an opportunity to do something constructive with the upcoming summer other than sleeping until 2:00 PM most days. I mailed the application for the program and received an invitation to the audition, which was held in Albany, NY. My father and I drove from Long Island to Albany where I successfully auditioned for the program. The audition committee consisted of just one man and he had extremely encouraging things to say after I played. From that point on I was excited about discovering the magic of the cello for the first time in my life.

When I arrived in Saratoga in August 1975, it was the turning point in my life. This was where I heard the Philadelphia Orchestra perform for the first time. The concert was at the outdoor Saratoga Performing Arts Center, and I still remember that magnificent Philadelphia sound. It was superior to anything I had ever heard and it was so rich and vibrant, I could almost see colors in the sounds. Over the next four weeks I was exposed to so much great music for the first time. The School of Orchestral Studies orchestra was at a far higher level than any of my previous musical experiences. I learned so much during those four weeks, but the true game changer was my two private lessons with the Philadelphia Orchestra's principal cellist William Stokking.

"In life, don't let people tell you what you can't do."

- William Stokking

The School of Orchestral Studies program included two cello sectionals each week, and the cellists in the program were extremely fortunate to have William Stokking as the instructor. At one of the cello sectionals, Mr. Stokking was going over the music with us and he noticed I was not paying attention. He became very angry and started yelling at me in front of all the other students. It was such an awful feeling. At the conclusion of the sectional, I approached Mr. Stokking with a humble apology, but he showed no interest in frivolous lip service. He did however take the time for a long talk, and said if I focused and worked hard, I could be a very accomplished cellist. From that moment, I decided to commit my entire life to the cello with no holds barred.

Upon returning home from Saratoga at the end of August, I phoned The Juilliard School about their pre-college program on Saturdays. They still had a cello opening and said I was welcome to come and audition. For the audition, I played music I had worked on with Mr. Stokking that summer, and I was accepted, however it was no time for celebration. Only seven months remained before upcoming conservatory auditions the following spring, and the Juilliard upper division was one of the four schools on my list. Needless to say, the following seven months were devoted exclusively to practicing the cello and preparing for auditions. The basement of the house became my private practice room, and on numerous occasions my mother came down at 2:00 AM to tell me it was time to stop practicing and go to bed because I had school the next day. Most times, I just said, "Mom, I have a lot of work to do. Please close the door behind you."

That hard work paid off because in the spring of 1976, I was accepted into The Juilliard School. However, showing up at Juilliard on the first day proved to be a sobering experience. Hearing all the other cellists play made me realize I was clearly out of my league, and I was one of the worst cellists in the school. I had almost no technical foundation on the instrument and knew close to nothing of the cello repertoire. Naturally, I was placed in the Conducting Orchestra, which was considered the entry-level group, and it is appropriately named because it is the orchestra in which the student conductors cut their teeth. At the first orchestra rehearsal, we played the Carnival Overture by Antonín Dvořák, and this work is taken at a very fast tempo. Not only was I not able to play the notes, but the music went by so fast my eyes were unable to even follow the music.

To make matters worse, about two weeks into that first year I attended a student recital at Juilliard by Charles Curtis, who was also a first-year cello student. Hearing him play was a rude awakening. He played at an extraordinarily high level and sounded more like an accomplished artist than a student. It is one thing to be the best in your high school or town, but Juilliard is a gathering of aspiring young people who are all the very best in their high schools and towns. As I sat listening to someone my age who played beautifully and was so many years ahead of me, I realized how far behind I was and how utterly impossible it would be to compete with people at this level. After the recital, I wanted to give up, and I had thoughts of stopping at a gun shop on the way home to quickly end my misery. The prospect of becoming an accomplished cellist now seemed unrealistic and insurmountable.

I had disadvantages, and the biggest was my first private cello teacher. Dorothy Bennert, who was the string teacher at my elementary school where I started playing the cello, called my mother after I had been playing for one year and said it was time for a private cello teacher. Since we lived so far out on Long Island in that "asshole of the world," the only choice for a local private cello teacher was a man who was vice president of a local savings bank, and not a professional cellist. Needless to say he was not an accomplished instrumentalist or teacher, but my mother liked him and he even came to our house for lessons.

Several days after that demoralizing recital by Charles Curtis, my luck changed when a violinist at Juilliard invited me to his apartment for a social hangout. It was an evening I will never forget because he played recordings by the violinist Jascha Heifetz. I had never heard a recording of his playing before. It was utterly amazing because his playing was absolutely flawless in every respect, and this was a level of string playing I had never before imagined. The following day I went to the Juilliard library to research Heifetz and find some answers to his ability to play an instrument at such an impossible level. After digging around, I found *The Way They Play*, Volume I, by Samuel Appelbaum, which is a compilation of interviews with the best string players of the time. It happened to include an extensive interview with Heifetz himself. In the book Heifetz offers advice to aspiring string players, and that advice transformed my approach to the cello.

In the interview, Heifetz is candid about the tendency of students in America to jump ahead to playing concertos without the necessary technical foundation. He stresses the critical importance of a solid technical foundation on the violin, which in his opinion is only achievable with the practice of scales. When Heifetz refers to scales, he means not only the common scale, but scales in all forms including arpeggios and the double stops, which are two notes played at once. Heifetz then changed my life with his recommendation for a student lacking a solid technical foundation. "I earnestly mean this. I would have him practice about three-fourths of his time on scales, and with it I would incorporate the other various weaknesses he may have."

This was exactly what I needed. I now had the master as my personal guide to help accomplish what I had set out to do with the cello. Though Heifetz was a violinist, I knew the basic principles of playing the violin and cello were the same. Patelson Music House was located on 56th Street directly behind Carnegie Hall. This was the world famous place to find sheet music and it was where one would often run into some of the world's greatest classical musicians. It was here I found a scale book for the cello that was so extensive, it seemed like Heifetz himself had written it.

The following day I brought the scale book to my cello lesson and informed my teacher, Channing Robbins, that I wanted to spend "three-fourths of my time on scales" while working from this book. He was concerned about this approach, which he considered radical. He said it was equally important to learn etudes and cello repertoire in addition to scales, but he compromised and agreed to help me with the scales if I promised to spend no more than one-third of my practice time on them. After agreeing to the terms, I went back to my apartment and got busy practicing scales. My threefold strategy was to initially focus almost exclusively on scales, which is cello technique in its simplest form. Then the emphasis would progress to etudes, which are short musical pieces based on specific technical concepts. When a technical foundation began to solidify, the focus would finally move to the cello repertoire, which would be learned at a much faster pace.

Adding to the problem of a deficient technical foundation was my bow arm, which desperately needed help, so my bow arm received some rather intensive attention for an extended period as well. The next day I passed a sidewalk sale near my apartment, and there was a large rectangular mirror in a heavy wooden frame offered for ten dollars. This seemed like the perfect teacher for a bow arm that was so bad it was causing pain in my right shoulder and neck. In my studio apartment, the mirror was set up on a chair opposite my practice chair, so it could assume the role of the bow-arm watchdog. For the better part of that first year I spent one full hour each morning in front of that mirror practicing only open strings. While practicing, I analyzed the details and timing of arm movement and continually searched for improvements of the bow grip.

As the year progressed it was becoming clear I was on the right track because I was making rapid improvement, and in the process, I was shedding the self-imposed reputation as one of the worst cellists at Juilliard. My progress was going as planned but the focus on the development of my technical foundation was still in its infancy, so the decision was made to devote the coming summer to the scale work. At the end of my first year at Juilliard, I locked myself in the apartment for the better part of that summer and practiced scales for no less than five hours every day, heeding Heifetz's recommendation of spending three-fourths of my time on scales. In addition to spending five hours every day on just scales, I devoted two hours to the cello etudes by David Popper, which are fiendishly difficult and widely considered to be the bible of the cello. Then the final two hours of each day were devoted to technically oriented literature written by some of the great cellists of the past.

Those intensive nine-hour practice days were one of the single wisest investments of my life. At the end of that summer, I had gained a technical proficiency on the cello that was propelling me past many of my Julliard colleagues who had been far ahead of me less than one year earlier. Two years later, I accidently bumped into the mirror that had been balancing on a chair all that time, and it hit the floor and smashed into pieces. I did not receive seven years of bad luck, but I will always miss that mirror because it was a great teacher and it gave a lifetime of good luck.

The obsessive and disciplined work on the cello led to the accomplishment of something that once seemed unachievable, but I was now faced with MS and it was time to start from ground zero once again. I had devoted everything I was capable of to learning the cello, but the current challenge would be far more difficult and would require double the effort. There were no method books for beating MS, and Jascha Heifetz would not be there to serve as my guide for building the technical foundation to beat the disease. This was not a challenge to learn a skill on a musical instrument; this was a situation where the stakes were much higher. There was no alternative career or backup plan if this failed. This was not about the cello, but a contest where the winner would take all. It was about beating an incurable illness and making a total recovery. I had taught myself how to play the cello, but now it was time to teach myself something infinitely more difficult.

Chapter 14

Several Crucial Findings

The Water Cure - "Why didn't I think of that?"

When I first got serious researching and understanding how to fight MS, I stumbled upon a website that offered one very simple and obvious solution. In life, the best inventions and discoveries are often the ones that are right there under our noses. Oftentimes it seems the sharpest minds will search for but overlook the most obvious answers, and then someone with relatively little experience happens to make the lucky discovery. From then on, everyone asks, "Why didn't I think of that?" The Water Cure belongs in this category because it is so basic that any child could have thought of it. Water is the basic necessity for life and the human body is mostly water. All parts of the body depend on water to function and this includes the circulatory, respiratory and the digestive systems. Our bodies need water for every single function including the elimination of human waste. However, in the case of MS the most important system of the body that depends on water to function is the central nervous system.

The website (*www.watercure.com*) is a condensed summary of the book *Your Body's Many Cries for Water* by Dr. F. Batmanghelidj. Using only water as a cure is beautiful because there is no financial incentive, and all special interests are removed from the equation. In his studies Dr. Batmanghelidj documents people with various chronic illnesses who improved dramatically just by following his easy formula of drinking water. It is unrealistic to foresee the insurance, pharmaceutical or medical industries rallying behind this approach, but perhaps the bottled water industry will. When a medical professional passionately promotes a remedy that has no profit motive, it deserves some attention.

The human body is mostly water, and the blood is 92 percent water. The blood is responsible for supplying oxygen and nutrients to the brain as well as all the other organs and tissues. Finding the Water Cure was a major piece of the puzzle and my only regret is not having known about it while on those insane doses of steroids earlier that year. Ironically, when I discovered the Water Cure in 1999, I was guided only by information that was available on the website. It would be several years before I would read the book. While the website offers the basic and helpful ideas, there is a great deal of information available only in the book. Therefore it is a must read for anyone with any kind of illness and for anyone who will deal with an illness in the future – that means everyone.

To summarize, Dr. Batmanghelidj's recommendation is simple: multiply half your body weight in pounds by one ounce of water. This number, in ounces, is the minimum daily intake of water. For example, I weigh 160 pounds, so my minimum intake of water is 80 ounces per day. When following this formula, it is important to drink only water; other liquids do not count. Diuretics such as alcohol, and caffeinated drinks such as coffee, tea, and energy drinks actually work to counter the benefits of the Water Cure by dehydrating the body. Juices, carbonated drinks, and even herbal tea should not be included as part of the formula.

I have no doubt the Water Cure was one of the most important weapons in my arsenal because I adhered to and exceeded the recommended formula with discipline, and I noticed improvement immediately. In addition to research and statistics, I began understanding the art of listening to my body. I learned to recognize the signs of bodily happiness as well as bodily complaints. One way the body signals a need for hydration is with a dry mouth, but few people seem to listen to this important communication. If the mouth is dry, it means hydration is inadequate and overdue. I do not wait until my mouth sends a dry signal, because that means the mouth is not the only part of the body that needs water. If the body becomes sufficiently hydrated regularly, it will grow accustomed to the fulfillment, and it will voice subtle complaints until its needs are met.

Many years ago when the Philadelphia Orchestra toured Israel, there was a free day when we could swim in the Dead Sea and climb Masada. The climb up Masada is a 45-minute workout in hot desert conditions. It is only for people in good physical condition and our tour guide warned us in advance to use the color of our urine as a guide. He stressed that our urine should be clear, and a yellow color meant we were inadequately hydrated. I put this useful tip to use years later when I began the Water Cure.

I quickly noticed the benefits of hydrating the body to an almost radical degree. There was immediate improvement in every part of my body, particularly the places that MS had hit the hardest. It may be a coincidence, but my eyes, hands and strength all began improving around the time I began the Water Cure. That led to my own belief that MS is exacerbated by an overheated central nervous system, and water will literally act as the fire extinguisher.

In light of the initial improvement, I began substantially exceeding the minimum water intake recommendation, and during hot weather, I doubled the amount. Within a short time, I was drinking 64 ounces every morning before any food, even before leaving the house for the orchestra rehearsals. After drinking one-half gallon of water, the feeling of hunger would not surface for several hours, and I felt a dramatic increase in energy and stamina from sufficiently hydrating my body.

Consuming that amount of water every morning posed major challenges during the orchestra rehearsals because the first break of the morning rehearsal took place after 75 long uncomfortable minutes. After 64 ounces of water, postponing that bio-break for one hour and fifteen minutes often proved difficult, but over time, I learned to train the bladder to accommodate the schedule. Leaving the stage during an orchestra rehearsal is awkward, but leaving the stage during an orchestra concert is taboo unless there is a legitimate emergency. For this reason the lion's share of my hydration takes place in the morning, and I am always careful to not over-hydrate before an evening concert. Drinking such a large amount of water in the morning will initially be an unpleasant experience but it is part of the discipline required to beat an incurable illness.

One modification I made to Dr. Batmanghelidj's formula was to eliminate his recommendation of adding one-quarter teaspoon of sea salt to each quart (32 ounces) of water consumed. Sodium is essential for the human body, but most people greatly exceed their needed intake of sodium. One-quarter teaspoon of salt is 590 mg of sodium, and if I followed Dr. Batmanghelidj's recommendation of adding salt to my 80 ounces per day, it would mean a daily dose of 1475 mg of sodium. That would be my daily dose of sodium only from the water, without any consideration for what is in food. I have learned to listen to my body, and it communicates an extremely small need for salt and loudly protests when its basic sodium requirement is exceeded.

I happen to have arthritis in only one place of my body, which is the base of my right big toe. Several years ago, the joint began swelling, and after having an x-ray of the joint, the radiologist concluded it was degenerative joint disease (DJD), the medical terminology for arthritis. I have had this condition for more than twenty years, but it is kept in check by restricting my salt intake. One welcome side effect of having this isolated case of arthritis is the early warning sentinel that is activated when excess salt is present in my system. While eating a meal with excess salt, I actually feel pain in the swollen toe joint before the meal is finished. If I consume too much salt, I am able to calm matters and quell the body's protests by drinking extra water to flush out the salt. It requires several hours for the rinse cycle to finish, but it effectively rids my body of the excess salt.

Many people may not have the same benefits of their arthritis acting as a salt alarm but there are other ways the body communicates high levels of salt. The morning after a high salt meal is the time the body will protest with noticeably swollen fingers, tight rings and puffy eyes. This is a perfect moment to rectify the ingestion of an unhealthy meal by having one liter of water for breakfast. One unforeseen benefit of following the Water Cure turned out to be the reduced intake of food, which means a reduced caloric intake and a subsequent loss of excess body weight. Drinking half of one's body weight in ounces is a substantial amount of water, and that leaves less room in the stomach for food. The Water Cure is a much easier and safer way of shedding weight than a gastrointestinal bypass.

Many feel strongly that one should eat first thing in the morning, but I refrain from eating until my body communicates a need for food. The only time I eat in the morning before feeling hunger is before a long bike ride or hike. Generally, my first sensation of hunger happens around noon, which also happens to be right around the time of the orchestra rehearsal break.

Several days after discovering the Water Cure, the website disappeared and there was no way to access it. I assumed this was a conspiracy by the pharmaceutical industry because they saw the Water Cure as a threat and had it blocked. However, one day later I was proven wrong when the website was back up and running. My updated theory was now a reverse conspiracy by the bottled water industry that got the website back online.

I will forever believe in the Water Cure and even though I have beaten MS, I continue to adhere to a daily intake of at least 80 ounces of water. I always carry one or two one-liter (33.814 ounce) stainless steel water bottles with me, and each day begins by drinking at least one liter before consuming any food. Even at the airport where bringing water through security is no longer permitted, I carry along a portable water filter that always sets off bells at the TSA X-ray machine. After successfully evading confiscation of the water filter, I head to an airport water fountain and filter two to three liters of water depending on the length of the flight. It is a documented fact that flying in an artificially dry and pressurized cabin of an aircraft efficiently dehydrates the body. Combine that with sitting in a small seat for many hours without being able to move, and it can lead to blood clots and other related problems. Therefore, increased water intake is compulsory before, during and after flying. Once again, keep in mind alcohol and caffeinated drinks such as coffee and tea, will actually worsen dehydration.

The Philadelphia Orchestra's flights to Asia can be as long as fifteen hours, so before one of these marathon flights, I consume three to four liters of water. That may sound extreme, but during the long flights, my body and state of mind do express their appreciation. If one drinks such large amounts of water before flying, it would be prudent to reserve an aisle seat so repeated requests to be excused from a window or middle seat do not make one an unpopular traveler. Assigning top credit to any single source in my victory against MS is impossible, but the Water Cure belongs right up there. This is simplicity at its best, for there are no copays, no prior insurance approvals and no fossil fuel burning trips to the drugstore. It should be made clear that the Water Cure worked for me, but caution should be used to avoid drinking too much water. I will once again stress how this book only details what I did to beat MS, and there is no promise or guarantee that the steps I took will work for other people. MS affects everyone differently therefore people should consult with their neurologist, do their own research and make their own decisions. A segment of the medical community has also raised valid questions about Dr. Batmanghelidj's studies. Most research and clinical trials are controlled studies that are subject to independent review. There are apparent reservations about Dr. Batmanghelidj's studies due to his alleged uncontrolled study procedures. Despite all of his doubters, I am grateful to have discovered the writings of Dr. Batmanghelidj. I will always believe the Water Cure was one of the key factors in my successful battle against MS.

Hydrating Nature's Cooling System

Sweating during exercise and particularly in hot weather requires a great deal of water. Therefore, water intake should be increased proportionately so fluid is not pilfered from the central nervous system and the regular functioning of the body. To drink so much water one must plan because society has become a place where the public toilet has gone the way of the dinosaur. Timing is everything in life, and planning for adequate water consumption requires timing. During the Philadelphia Orchestra's summer season, concerts take place at the Mann Center in Philadelphia's Fairmount Park and at the Saratoga Performing Arts Center in Saratoga Springs, NY, where the heat and humidity are often oppressive. The orchestra also plays a July series in Vail, CO, which hosts a potentially hazardous combination of an altitude of 8,120 feet (2,475 meters) with extremely low humidity. In this mountain environment the body will not visibly perspire as profusely as it does in the hot humid Philadelphia summer, so it is easy to be misled by an apparent lack of sweat. In such a high and dry environment, the body will require just as much water as it does in a hot and humid one.

I manage to play these outdoor summer concerts by consuming half a liter of water just before the concert begins, and at intermission of the concert, I am the first one in the men's room. Prior to the second half of the concert, I drink another half-liter and relieve myself one last time before the second half begins. The challenge of drinking so much water while performing with a symphony orchestra is when we play those ninety-minute symphonies of Gustav Mahler. We play these lengthy masterworks without a break, but I have luckily made it this far without having to leave the stage during a concert. The difficulties of performing in hot humid summer concerts are not only compounded by hot stage lighting, but also by the acoustic shells around the stage, which limit airflow and can act as a heat retainer. During every summer concert, a water bottle always hides by my side as an emergency backup in the event a dry mouth should show its face.

Chronic Illness and Exercise

One early helpful find was an article in the *Journal of American Medicine and Sports,* and it would prove to be another game changer that helped change a pessimistic outlook to one of optimism. The article stressed the importance of exercise for people with chronic illnesses as well as for people in perfect health. There is a natural tendency for people diagnosed with MS to curtail and even avoid exercise. This temptation is understandable because it can easily stem from the fear of another exacerbation. There was no medical breakthrough with the article and the best part was its simplicity. It is basic common sense and anyone could have thought of it. The article was an important step forward because it provided me with an early sign of hope. I even went one step further and began searching for possible links not only between MS and a lack of physical fitness, but also MS and an unhealthy diet and questionable lifestyle.

Rates of MS in Japan

Looking at worldwide rates of MS was helpful, but the big surprise was the low occurrence of MS in Asian countries. Japan in particular stood out because it is located on the same latitude as the northeastern United States, but the occurrence of MS in Japan is very low. It is no exaggeration to say Japan has serious environmental issues, and overcrowding there has to be seen to be believed. Japan squeezes the equivalent of nearly half the population of the United States into an area the size of Wyoming.

What were the reasons for much lower rates of MS? The first and most obvious thing that came to mind is diet. The typical Japanese diet differs dramatically from the Western diet because it is largely comprised of rice, fish and vegetables, and the portions are far smaller. While many traditional Japanese dishes may strike some Westerners as a meal that "washed up on the beach," the all too common U.S. diet consists of massive amounts of meat and dairy, along with processed foods.

Since joining the Philadelphia Orchestra in 1985, I have been on each of the orchestra's tours of Japan. In 1997 when I took a sabbatical from the orchestra, I toured Japan for two weeks as a substitute cellist with the Baltimore Symphony. On my first visit to Japan, I was treated to a lavish dinner in one of Tokyo's most exclusive restaurants, and one of the first items served was a bowl of whale soup. I stared at the soup pondering if it was the appropriate moment to stage a protest or to remain silent and eat the soup. I reluctantly decided to assume the role of a polite guest, so I forced down the soup which I admit tasted good but it was extra heavy on the guilt. Eating that bowl of soup haunts me to this day because it is difficult to comprehend the necessity of killing a whale to make soup. For the next course two delicacies were presented, a gigantic live shrimp and a live octopus. The shrimp was cut in half right at the table, and then the live head was placed on a plate, complete with moving eyes and antennae. I sat there contemplating eating something that was looking back at me with moving eyes, but I was unable to bring myself to do so. Next was the live octopus. The tentacles were cut off right at the table and once again placed on a plate for immediate consumption. When I attempted to pick up a moving tentacle with a pair of chopsticks, it was difficult because the suction cups were tenaciously gripping the surface of the plate. After a moment I managed to get the upper hand on the severed arm and proceeded to place it in my mouth. One of the strangest moments in all my dining experiences was when octopus suction cups were grabbing my tongue and the roof of my mouth. Putting something in one's mouth that is moving might be good during an intimate and passionate moment with someone special, but if it is a live creature of the sea the experience will definitely take some getting used to. The definite bright side of the previous two dishes is the lack of processing involved. This was certainly food in its most natural state.

The Okinawa Centenarian Study

I happened to find the Okinawa Centenarian Study while looking for statistical occurrences of MS in the world. The amazing part of this was not just the low rate of MS in Japan, but Okinawa in particular where the rate of MS in the group studied was unheard of. The Okinawa Centenarian Study (OCS) is an extensive and detailed study of more than 900 Okinawans that were all over the age of 100. MS was not the only rarity in the study, but many other common illnesses were rarities as well. Incredibly, the women from the study have never been screened for ovarian or cervical cancer because the occurrences of these diseases are so rare amongst people in this study. Amongst the men, there were almost no recorded cases of prostate cancer. Many of our trademark ailments in the West, such as heart disease, high blood pressure, type 2 diabetes, rheumatism and obesity were almost nonexistent in this group.

The Okinawa diet is vegetable and grain based, but a significant difference from the Western diet is the size of the portions. The study subjects ate until they were only eighty-percent full; as opposed to the Western practice of eating until the stomach is overloaded to the point breathing normally becomes a challenge. The typical OCS diet does include meat, but when meat is on the menu the portion is limited to the size of a deck of playing cards. It is ironic the former reigning competitive eating champion Takeru Kobayashi is a native of Japan, but I doubt anyone in the OCS would have been a formidable challenger in the annual Nathan's Famous Hot Dog Eating Contest, which takes place every year in Coney Island, NY. I wonder how many participants in that competitive eating event will go on to be centenarians.

The authors of the OCS tend to emphasize genetics as a main reason for longevity, but I believe lifestyle is a far more important factor. We cannot change our genetic makeup but we can definitely change our lifestyle. The OCS convinced me that overeating is one of the worst things for the body, and I also believe overeating efficiently negates any benefit of healthy eating. After studying the OCS, I strongly believe reducing caloric intake is one of the single most important factors for a long and healthy life. However, my problem was not to stay healthy, it was to get healthy. Getting healthy was first on the list and nothing was going to stop me from reaching that goal. If I found what it would take to get healthy and continued the practice, then staying healthy would be easy.

All You Can Eat

A man walks into a restaurant that displays a sign advertising "All You Can Eat." He fills a plate at the buffet table then sits down and has a few bites, and suddenly a big guy comes out and says, "That's all you can eat. Now get out!"

I love this joke because "all you can eat" stands alone as a hilarious concept. We may feel economically savvy by getting a big bang for the buck at one of the many all you can eat restaurants, but the resulting excess caloric intake risks delivering a big bang full of buck (as in buckshot). It is commonly accepted that overeating reduces the lifespan of mice, rats and rabbits and even fruit flies. I know dog owners who feed their dogs an exclusive diet of dry dog food; they swear it keeps their dogs both trim and living a longer, healthier life. Dry dog food cannot be very exciting to the canine palate, but dogs that live on dry kibble will tend to eat just enough to quell their hunger. The likely explanation of the longevity of dogs that live exclusively on dry food is their reduced caloric intake. The more I looked at the benefits of reduced caloric intake, the more it made perfect sense.

In the United States a normal portion of food is enough for four or five people, which is far more calories than the body is able to handle. Therefore, when excess calories are consumed, the body is presented with the challenge of how to deal with the excess. Among the many unwelcome consequences of overeating is the release of free radicals, or unstable molecules within the system, and as a result, the body is prone to numerous ailments. After considering that, I began looking at the possible links between overeating and many common ailments, including MS. The common Western ailments of today are nothing new, but the current epidemic rates of some of those ailments are unprecedented.

Do Not Feed the Deer

In 1985 while on a backpacking trip in Shenandoah National Park, Virginia, I noticed a sign outside a Visitor Center with a picture of a deer and a warning: "DO NOT FEED THE DEER. When you feed a deer human food such as chips and candy, you reduce its lifespan by 30%." If only I had captured a photo of that moment.

Is it realistic to believe the human body will remain unaffected by chips and candy? Are we physiologically so different from deer that our bodies will handle junk food with no ill effects? Have we blindly accepted a reduced lifespan that is caused by an unhealthy diet and lifestyle as an acceptable cost of doing business? Would we live longer and healthier if we followed the dietary practice of a deer? If so, living on such a diet would essentially mean drinking only water and eating only natural raw food.

Humans are a funny species. We do certain things to an extreme degree while we neglect some of the vitally important things that need attention, and our bodies are a perfect example. We treat our hair to the best designer shampoos, conditioners and styling gels. Our skin is pampered with natural soaps and treated with wonderful oils and lotions to restore its luster and beauty. Dental conditioning is seen to with Teflon coated flosses and toothbrushes that clean the teeth, and condition and massage the gums. Toothpaste is used to prevent tooth decay, to control tartar and whiten the teeth. Mouthwash is then used for conditioning of the breath. Many people even take gelatin to condition their fingernails. The list continues with products for just about every external part of the body.

With all the time, thought and resources that are devoted to caring for the exterior of the human body, relatively little is devoted to caring for the interior of the body. I personally know people who only fill the fuel tank of their car with premium gasoline, yet without a second thought they fill their bodies with junk food, alcohol and tobacco, which are damaging fuels for the mind as well as the body. When fighting MS it is important to remember the mind and body will have plenty to do just battling the disease. Distracting the mind and body with unhealthy food and drink places a person at a disadvantage when fighting MS, therefore to be a serious contender one must abstain from substances that can weaken the ability of the mind and body to fight.

Techno-Food

I grew up with 45 rpm and 33 rpm long-playing records, and later I saw the birth and death of the 8-track player. I saw the rise and fall of the cassette and the Sony Walkman, and now I am witnessing the end of the audio compact disk or CD. I even remember when the microwave became available for everyone and how this new and fascinating oven of the future could heat up food so quickly. Technology has advanced so far and produced so many wonderful things that make this a truly privileged age in which to live. We have sophisticated electronics and computers for transportation, work, home and play. It is now possible to be any place on the planet in twenty-four hours. Heart transplants will soon be rendered obsolete by battery-powered pumps, and it will not be long before cars drive themselves. With each passing day, life is moving ahead and changing at an ever-faster pace.

One major downside to these technological advances is the loss of simplicity in our diet. I refer to today's Western diet as techno-food because it is designed in a laboratory, approved by a board of directors, grown from genetically modified organisms and made in a mass production factory. The shareholders are the driving force behind the food; the consumer's health and well-being are secondary. This modern high tech diet is unprecedented and foreign to our bodies because our meals contain large amounts of fat, salt, sugar, processed food, chemical preservatives, along with artificial coloring and flavoring. Coffee, alcohol, energy drinks and soda sweetened with inexpensive high fructose corn syrup have replaced water to meet our hydration needs. The standard unbalanced Western diet is often heavy on meat and dairy, while light on vegetables and grains. "All You Can Eat" restaurants are all the rage, where people gorge themselves with plate after plate. A sedentary lifestyle works in tandem with an unbalanced diet to form a launch pad for a plethora of Western diseases. I have little doubt that rheumatism, gout, arthritis, type 2 diabetes, high blood pressure, high cholesterol, and MS are largely caused by poor dietary and lifestyle choices. Many will disagree that MS belongs in this group, but there is one study that should be considered:

The World Health Organization and The Multiple Sclerosis International Federation published Atlas - Multiple Sclerosis Resources in the World 2008. This study has limits because some countries did not respond to the survey on rates of MS, but it is still worth a look. Globally, the median estimated prevalence of MS is 30 cases per 100,000 people. By income category, the median estimated prevalence of MS is greatest in high-income countries (89 MS cases per 100,000 people), followed by upper middle income (32 MS cases per 100,000 people), and lower middle and low-income countries (10 MS cases per 100,000 people). The total estimated number of people diagnosed with MS, reported by the countries that responded, is 1,315,579 of whom approximately 630,000 are in Europe, 520,000 in the Americas, 66,000 in the Eastern Mediterranean, 56,000 in the Western Pacific, 31,500 in South East Asia and 11,000 in Africa.

I am not a scientist, doctor, nutritionist or a statistician, so my research focused on finding obvious things that may have been overlooked by those experts. I looked for answers that would be followed up with "Why didn't I think of that?" It would be difficult to debate that wealthy societies tend to indulge in a rich lavish diet, while poorer nations do not. After considering these MS rates around the world, I began crafting a plan to live on a low-income diet by eating very simple food and reducing the size of my portions. Keep in mind that deer from Shenandoah National Park did not live on a high-income diet.

The Natural Diet of Man

The Natural Diet of Man is a chapter in *The Complete Illustrated Book of Yoga*, by Swami Vishnudevananda, and it is one of the best yoga books ever written on the subject. I discovered this book as a teenager many years before

I was diagnosed with MS, and my initial draw to this book was to increase the flexibility in my legs. The yoga poses were very helpful for my tight hamstrings, but the chapter titled "The Natural Diet of Man" really caught my attention. After reading the chapter, I was so moved that I decided to stop eating meat. I subsequently embarked on a revolutionary vegetarian diet without giving much thought to my nutritional needs, so the new diet was highly unbalanced and undisciplined. That brainstorm diet lasted for a couple of years then I slowly began eating meat once again, but during my first year at Juilliard I discovered the world of macrobiotic food. A neighbor on the tenth floor of my apartment building showed me the basics of an organic and natural diet, and although I gravitated to this healthier and more balanced diet, I did not become disciplined about it until my bout with MS years later. "The Natural Diet of Man" chapter is not tailored to fighting MS because it includes a good amount of dairy, and I firmly believe dairy and MS do not mix. Seventy-five percent of the world's adult population does not drink milk, so I decided I would survive without dairy as well. Dairy is a large part of the diet in many of the wealthy industrialized nations, and this is where the rates of MS are higher. In order to rid my body of the disease, I decided to give up dairy and eat like a pauper.

The Portable Air Conditioner

In early July of 1999, I was on a personal mission to prove I had been misdiagnosed with MS, so I was engaging in those strenuous thirty-mile bike rides in the Catskill Mountains of upstate New York in the heat and humidity. Dr. Markowitz believes there is no definitive way of knowing if that intense cardio activity in the heat could have been responsible for the subsequent third attack, but I remain convinced there had to be some correlation. On the other hand, it is difficult to argue with Dr. Markowitz's opinions because he leaves little to guesswork, and I will always be thankful for his decision to put me on that 10-day radical dose of intravenous steroids. It was the right call.

In April 1999, Dr. Lublin advised avoiding exercise to the point of sweating, but I ignored his advice because I thought I knew better. There is a saying, "The baker eats his mistakes and the doctor buries his mistakes." Looking back on the decision to go on those monster bike rides in the heat before the big attack, I feel lucky not to have buried my own mistake. After things finally did calm down following my intense third MS attack, I was extremely careful not to overheat the body or stress the central nervous system in any way. During my first year of recovery, I kept my house temperature a cool 60 degrees Fahrenheit in the winter out of fear of overheating the body and subsequently suffering a dreaded fourth attack.

There are many theories about why the symptoms of MS tend to worsen in high heat and humidity. Much more is now known about the subject and recent studies have shown a direct correlation between heat and MS symptoms. One likely explanation for the link is damage to the myelin that protects the nerves. When the myelin is damaged the nerves are far more susceptible to even small changes in the temperature of the body's core. I wish I had heeded Dr. Lublin's advice to "not exercise to the point of sweating." Only after my third attack did I begin to act with caution and sensibility. If nothing was learned from the results of my 30-mile bicycle rides in the hills during a July heat wave, I would truly qualify as intellectually challenged. After the brutal 1999 attack I became a firm believer in the need to take every precaution against overheating. I did not research any possible relationship between MS and overheating after this but my theories and actions all stemmed from listening to my body. To say the heat worsened my symptoms in 1999 would be an understatement. Not only did it worsen my symptoms, it was as if I had been hit by a train.

Every species adapts to its surrounding environment, but humans are the only species that does not. Instead, we adapt our surrounding environment to suit our needs and desires. Many people with MS will restrict themselves to air conditioned environments during the summer months. This practice subjects a person to constant indoor air pollution, which should be a major concern for everyone. It not only limits fresh air, outdoor activity and exercise, but it also reduces exposure to some needed daily sunlight. I decided that MS would not stop me from working or engaging in outdoor activities, so the search was underway to find some way to keep the body cool while partaking in normal outdoor summer activities. The way humans adapt to their surrounding environment is by layering clothing in the winter and adequately hydrating in the summer. Unfortunately, there are limits to both approaches, particularly in the summer heat.

To regulate body temperature in a hot and humid environment, the body produces sweat, which cools the body by drawing away heat. The human body's cooling system is similar to an electric air conditioner in the sense it consumes energy and resources. During heat and humidity the human cooling system uses large amounts of water to produce sweat, and this water is provided to the sweat glands by the blood, which is 92 percent water. I strongly believe it is critically important to keep the body sufficiently hydrated during the initial year after being diagnosed; I looked for ways to stay cool by drawing as little water from the blood as possible.

One helpful solution was discovered when I read a book on backpacking. It was a cautionary measure against the cold. Wet cotton clothing during cold temperatures can be deadly as it efficiently steals body heat, creating an invitation for hypothermia. Backpackers have a motto: "Cotton kills." The summer is a great time for outdoor fun, but when people with MS engage in outdoor activities during hot humid weather, the potential for trouble exists.

The summer of 2000 was a hot one and I did not want to miss my son's Little League baseball games or give up my bike rides. Necessity is the mother of invention, so I came up with a way to stay cool out in the sun along with the heat and humidity. For the Little League games, I attended every one my schedule allowed by simply dressing for the part. Long sleeve white shirts and hats made of heavy cotton will hold a great deal of water, and a wet shirt and a wet hat will effectively draw heat from the body. This may be a winter recipe for disaster, but in the summer, it proved to be a godsend. I experimented with the concept of wet clothing and it worked even better than I had envisioned. The shirt and hat were soaked in water then wrung out only to the point they stopped dripping. Even in the hottest weather, a wet cotton shirt feels ice-cold going on, as it instantly becomes an efficient heat exchanger. What would be a quick death in the winter suddenly became an effective portable air conditioner in the summer.

That summer I resumed those long bike rides but now with the advantage of my new designer clothing line. It worked wonders and gave me a greater understanding of just how hard the body works to stay cool while exercising in hot humid conditions. Before coming down with MS the only way I knew to keep cool during previous bike rides was to drink more water, so this find was yet another piece of the puzzle that fell nicely into place. Even on long rides in temperatures of 95 degrees Fahrenheit, I was sweating far less with the wet cotton clothing than ever before because my body was no longer struggling to stay cool. When cycling in such weather, a heavy white cotton shirt will remain wet for 30 – 45 minutes, so several shirt-wetting stops became a regular part of my summer cycling. I always found places to wet my shirt such as a convenience store spigot, a lawn sprinkler or even a stream, so periodic rewetting of my shirt enabled me to ride for several hours with comfort. One additional and obvious benefit to a heavy long-sleeve white shirt is protection from the sun. Sunlight in small amounts is needed for good health but too much direct sunlight is definitely harmful for the skin. I always choose white shirts because the color white tends to reflect sunlight and heat, and that helps keep my body temperature cooler. A dark colored shirt actually absorbs sunlight and heat, and that works to raise the body temperature.

My stubborn mindset would not permit any cessation of cycling in the summer, so the clever and novel idea of riding with heavy wet clothing literally proved to be a life-saver. Staying sufficiently hydrated made even more sense as time progressed. Before every ride I overhydrated in advance and did not limit my cycling during hot weather. I guessed correctly because I never suffered another attack after 1999. I also took cooler showers during my recovery. Letting the water trickle allowed me to effectively clean my body and wash my hair with cool water. Rinsing the soap and shampoo took a bit longer than usual, but my body was not subjected to any sudden change in temperature.

I believe it is vital to take the first year after diagnosis very seriously because it can set the stage for years to come. For extended periods outside in the heat, I always plan to have access to a water source to keep my heavy cotton shirt wet. It is very important to adequately hydrate before heading out in the heat, so I make sure to carry extra water bottles as an emergency backup.

Chapter 15

A Declaration of War

The U.S. Army Survival Guide and the Psychology of Surviving and Beating an Illness

When I was initially diagnosed with MS, it was only a fight against a disease. Six months later I was fighting for my survival. To find ways to fight the disease, I cut to the chase and reduced the equation to its lowest common denominator. MS is an enemy that lies in wait, strikes without warning and withdraws back into hiding. This insurgent does not play by the rules; I could not fight by the rules. MS will surprise a person with creative and unexpected ways to attack; therefore, it is necessary to find creative and unexpected ways to fight back. This is guerilla warfare at its worst, so the battle cannot be fought only with the conventional weapons used to fight some other diseases.

Every year since 2003, I go on a September hiking trip with four of my buddies, and the tradition of these male-bonding trips is to visit a different National Park each year. One of my favorite things about this annual trip is the total void of alcohol. Three of the guys are friends of Bill (the not-so-secret code word for membership in a certain alcohol-free club), so there is no stopping at liquor stores or bars, and there is no social pressure to drink. Our past trips have included the Grand Canyon, Yellowstone, Glacier, Sequoia, Tetons, Denali and the Smoky Mountains. Because of the serenity and the sheer beauty of the surroundings, some of my best writing ideas came while hiking in the wilderness.

74

In 2013, we visited Crater Lake National Park in Oregon, then the Northern California Redwoods. On September 19, 2013, we had just hiked two and a half miles to a beautiful waterfall in the middle of the redwoods and my cell phone rang. Astonished there was reception in this remote location, I looked and saw the caller was an unknown four-digit number. I had a feeling it was a telemarketer but I answered it anyway, and lo and behold it was the United States Army John F. Kennedy Special Warfare Center and School in Fort Bragg, North Carolina. One week earlier, I mailed them a letter describing my situation, and requested permission to use passages from the *U.S. Army Survival Guide* in my book. The caller was a woman from the Commander's office and she was fascinated the *U.S. Army Survival Guide* was actually used to fight MS. Therefore permission was granted to reprint passages from the manual provided due credit was given.

I am no closet mercenary nor have I ever served in the armed forces, but I have always been fascinated with wilderness survival and the stories of those who survived life-threatening situations against impossible odds. Many years ago, before any hint of MS, I was bitten by the backpacking bug and I purchased several books on backpacking and wilderness survival, and one of them was the *U.S. Army Survival Guide*. I read the guide and put it away without realizing it would be stored in my subconscious for use years later.

This look at the *U.S. Army Survival Guide* will not deal with scorpion or snake bites, but that particular section of the guide might be helpful for any patients who may have overindulged in bee sting therapy. The part of the guide that applies to battling MS and other illnesses is purely psychological. When battling a disease such as MS it cannot be merely a fight against an illness, but it must be a fight for survival. In life threatening situations, the ones who survive are the ones with the right mindset. That mindset includes the will and spirit to live, the ability to never lose hope no matter how bleak the situation may be, the ability to overcome pain and discomfort, and the ability of the mind to supersede the limits of the human body.

The comparisons between wilderness survival and fighting MS are strikingly similar, and in the *U.S. Army Survival Guide,* one can frequently substitute MS for the words wilderness or hostile environment. Fighting MS requires thinking outside the box, connecting the dots and finding comparisons and analogies to use in battle. This guide is the perfect tool and companion for anyone diagnosed with the disease, as it is immeasurably helpful with planning and establishing the necessary fighting spirit.

The key paragraphs listed here are taken directly from the *U.S. Army Survival Guide*, and they will prove invaluable when battling an illness.

From Chapter 1:

Value Living

> *"All of us were born kicking and fighting to live, but we have become used to the soft life. We have become creatures of comfort. We dislike inconveniences and discomforts. What happens when we are faced with a survival situation with its stresses, inconveniences, and discomforts? This is when the will to live—placing a high value on living—is vital. The experience and knowledge you have gained through life and your Army training will have a bearing on your will to live. Stubbornness, a refusal to give in to problems and obstacles that face you, will give you the mental and physical strength to endure."*

From Chapter 2

Psychology of Survival

> *"Some people with little or no survival training have managed to survive life-threatening circumstances. Some people with survival training have not used their skills and died. A key ingredient in any survival situation is the mental attitude of the individual involved. Having survival skills is important; having the will to survive is essential. Without a desire to survive, acquired skills serve little purpose and invaluable knowledge goes to waste."*

Depression

> *"You would be a rare person indeed if you did not get sad, at least momentarily,*

when faced with the hardships of survival. As this sadness deepens, it becomes "depression." Depression is closely linked with frustration and anger. Frustration will cause you to become increasingly angry as you fail to reach your goals. If the anger does not help you succeed, then the frustration level goes even higher. A destructive cycle between anger and frustration will continue until you become worn down—physically, emotionally, and mentally. When you reach this point, you start to give up, and your focus shifts from "What can I do" to "There is nothing I can do." Depression is an expression of this hopeless, helpless feeling. There is nothing wrong with being sad as you temporarily think about your loved ones and remember what life is like back in "civilization" or "the world." Such thoughts, in fact, can give you the desire to try harder and live one more day. On the other hand, if you allow yourself to sink into a depressed state, then it can sap all your energy and, more important, your will to survive. It is imperative that you resist succumbing to depression."

Fear

"Fear is our emotional response to dangerous circumstances that we believe have the potential to cause death, injury, or illness. This harm is not just limited to physical damage; the threat to your emotional and mental well-being can generate fear as well. If you are trying to survive, fear can have a positive function if it encourages you to be cautious in situations where recklessness could result in injury. Unfortunately, fear can also immobilize you. It can cause you to become so frightened that you fail to perform activities essential for survival. Most people will have some degree

77

of fear when placed in unfamiliar surroundings under adverse conditions. There is no shame in this! You must train yourself not to be overcome by your fears. Ideally, through realistic training, you can acquire the knowledge and skills needed to increase your confidence and thereby manage your fears."

Fear is a natural emotion that exists in all of us. When I was first diagnosed with MS my state of denial was generated by an intense fear of the disease. I acted recklessly by going on those thirty-mile bike rides in the hills during the summer heat and humidity. Accepting my diagnosis at that time was not a possibility and I was out to prove it was a misdiagnosis. After my brutal third attack it was clear there was no misdiagnosis. I was deathly afraid of a dreaded fourth MS attack that was ready to strike at any time, and I was scared to do anything that could possibly set it in motion.

According to the *U.S. Army Survival Guide* fear can be harmful or deadly, but it can also be positive. If used in a positive way, fear can guide one to proceed with caution rather than recklessness. After my third attack it was clear I needed to better understand and come to terms with my fear so it could be channeled to a more cautionary approach.

The *U.S. Army Survival Guide* is a must-read because of the wealth of information that is incredibly helpful for dealing with overwhelming fear and anxiety that come with being diagnosed. The guide will also help one to view the disease as a textbook enemy. It helped me become a highly skilled and elusive target when I was alone in enemy territory without friendly troops for support. The single most helpful part of the guide is the emphasis to stay calm, assess the situation, devise a plan, and to never give up or lose hope.

Do Not Just Act the Role of the Warrior - Become the Warrior

A soldier going to battle is not just issued a rifle and sent on his way. The soldier undergoes many months of training to prepare for a war zone. The first step is the basic training to condition the soldier physically and mentally, and that is only the start. The soldier will train and prepare for capture, interrogation and torture, and will learn how to tolerate pain and suffering, and to not crack under pressure. There is intense competition and endless training for a soldier to achieve the elite status of the Delta Force or the Navy

Seals. The soldier will even study and learn the enemy's surroundings, language and lifestyle habits. Brutal training conditions the mind for extreme hardship and suffering, and it teaches one to remain calm during the worst imaginable conditions.

To beat a disease as tough as MS, one must do more than see a neurologist, begin the recommended medication, and follow up with monitoring and testing. It will take everything a person is capable of, physically, emotionally, intellectually, and spiritually. As someone who has beaten the disease, I will say it is not possible to cure other people, but I can only explain and demonstrate how I accomplished curing myself. The only possible way for other MS patients to accomplish what I have done is to devote everything they have to finding their own path. It is impossible to teach a person how to ride a bicycle because endless visual examples and explanations will never succeed. The aspiring young cyclist will understand what has been explained only when the coordination of balancing on two wheels is mastered. Battling MS will require a similar understanding, but on a much higher and demanding level.

To battle MS I became not just a soldier, I became an elite Delta Force and MS warrior! I studied the enemy's language, its patterns of attack and learned its vulnerabilities. I fought the war from an offensive position and I struck MS in its Achilles heel at the most unexpected moments. I vowed to endure hardship and suffering under the worst possible conditions, and to persevere and never again be on the defensive against this stealthy enemy.

History illustrates how the Israelis won the 1967 Yom Kippur war when they were so heavily outnumbered. The Israelis faced overwhelming odds in a war they should have lost, and this is yet one more example of an impossible accomplishment. In preparation for the war, the Israeli forces were supplied with a more than adequate water supply for battle in dessert conditions; the Egyptian forces were not. Postmortem analysis of the war revealed a large number of Egyptian solders died not from battle, but from severe dehydration. It is important to remember that proper hydration of the body is as critical when fighting MS as it is when fighting in the desert.

Chapter 16

Clinical Trials and the Placebo Effect

Approved and accepted rules of science govern our world, and harsh judgment often falls upon those who question those rules. Galileo's support of the theory of heliocentrism was considered too radical, and he paid a price for defying those accepted rules of his day. Western medicine is also based on approved and accepted rules, but in medicine, events often take place that defy the rules. The placebo effect, a phenomenon that science and medicine cannot explain, is a perfect example of this. This anomaly does not abide by any accepted set of rules, but instead it follows its own rules.

"I Follow My Own Rules." - **Claude Debussy**

As a student, the great French composer Claude Debussy was reprimanded by his disapproving musical composition instructor for going outside of the accepted norms. "Young man, what rules do you follow?" The young Debussy replied, "I follow my own rules." His teacher responded, "That is alright, provided you are a genius."

The widely accepted approach to treating MS is to begin taking the latest drug with the hope of slowing the progression of the disease and the goal of getting and keeping it in remission. A common mindset is to then wait for the pharmaceutical industry to develop new and better drugs to arrest and actually reverse the disease. In his book, *Your Body's Many Cries for Water*, Dr. Batmanghelidj argues that the economy of the entire medical industry depends on the status quo of our current health care system. He points out there is a large amount of money at stake and the beneficiaries of this system include pharmaceutical companies, hospitals, doctors, nurses, makers of medical devices, health insurance companies, and particularly the government which generates income in the form of corporate and employee tax revenue. Even the Food and Drug Administration (FDA) is a beneficiary of this system as it is largely funded by fees from the very drug companies it is charged to oversee and regulate.

Rather than dwell on the shortcomings of our medical system, my focus remained on finding ways to fight MS that had been overlooked. When new drugs are developed and tested to fight various illnesses, placebo groups are part of most clinical trials. Surprisingly, researchers often ignore the inexplicable success in these groups. It is important to explore every possible reason behind the mystery instead of just dismissing it as an anomaly. I brought up this subject with Dr. Markowitz and asked for his opinion of the reason behind the placebo effect. He explained his theory that the brain produces a chemical that makes physical changes to the body. Some people believe God heals people through prayer. Yogis believe spiritual and mental development empowers the body to heal itself.

After researching the placebo effect, I became a firm believer that the mind can be trained to effectively make physical changes to the body. This is an ability we all possess to some degree. In a medical crisis, it is crucial to focus this skill toward fighting the illness. The process of training the mind to make changes in the body will come easily to some, while others will find it painstakingly difficult. When starting out to develop and empower the mind to heal the body, it is important to remember that the journey of a thousand miles begins with a single step. A positive attitude is compulsory and if one does not believe in the placebo effect, it will never work.

The concept of learning the placebo effect originally came after reading the package insert included with the monthly injection kit of Avonex®. I had been on this drug for several months but had never taken the time to read that long and involved fact sheet. One rainy day I sat down and went through the package insert, and I was startled to see statistics on the subjects in the clinical trial. The one statistic that caught my attention was the number of exacerbations after two years on Avonex®.

There were 301 subjects (patients) enrolled in the Avonex® clinical trial. Of the 301 subjects, 172 completed the two-year trial. Of the 172 subjects that completed the Avonex® clinical trial, 87 subjects were given a placebo, and 85 were given Avonex®.

The number of exacerbations (attacks or flare ups) in subjects that completed the two-year study.	Placebo (Total number of subjects = 87)	Avonex® (Total number of subjects = 85)
0 Exacerbations	23 out of 87 subjects	32 out of 85 subjects
1 Exacerbation	26 out of 87 subjects	26 out of 85 subjects
2 Exacerbations	10 out of 87 subjects	15 out of 85 subjects
3 Exacerbations	12 out of 87 subjects	6 out of 85 subjects
4 Exacerbations	16 out of 87 subjects	6 out of 85 subjects

After reading these numbers, I focused on the success rate of the placebo group that suffered only one exacerbation in the two-year study (26 out of 87 on the placebo vs. 26 out of 85 on the Avonex®). This success of both of these groups was nearly identical, so I began looking at other MS drug trials and cases where the placebo groups achieved high success rates.

When a pharmaceutical company develops a new drug, it cannot be sold in the U.S. unless the FDA has approved it for sale. The FDA will approve a drug only after it has been subjected to rigorous testing and has successfully passed each of those tests. Coincidentally, my wife Teresa whom I met after my recovery, is a lead clinical research associate with a major pharmaceutical company. My education in clinical trials took place at the end of each day when I asked Teresa how her workday went. Teresa shared stories about the day while somehow assuming I was familiar with all the terminology used in clinical trials. To maintain a successful marriage it is important for one to be a good listener, so I made it a point of learning the language to have a better idea of what my wife was saying without constantly interrupting the conversation with requests for definitions. Initially I did not understand the clinical trial lingo, but as I gained knowledge on the subject, it gave me a clear understanding of what I had accomplished with the help of the placebo effect. It not only gave a clearer understanding of what I had accomplished with the help of the placebo effect, it also made me a better listener and husband.

When delving into general research on MS trials, I found that the disproportionately high success rate among subjects in the placebo groups posed a challenge unique to MS trials. It was surprising to see the medical community and the pharmaceutical industry overlook this rate of success. There had to be answers within this mystery, so I became almost obsessed with the subject and began looking into this accepted anomaly. For those who believe there are no answers in the success of clinical trial placebo groups, one needs only to look at the Rogaine® clinical trial study, and particularly the placebo group in that trial. Rogaine® or the generic equivalent minoxidil is a drug for treating hair loss.

Early in my recovery, I had an appointment with my dermatologist Warren S. Kurnick, in Willingboro, NJ, for a case of poison ivy, which resulted from clearing brush out of my back yard. Years earlier, Dr. Kurnick earned my complete trust and respect because of an incident involving a rather large sebaceous cyst on my scalp. A sebaceous cyst is a benign growth that supposedly originates from a clogged hair follicle. In my case they may be hereditary because my father was also prone to them.

Years before I knew Dr. Kurnick, my family doctor recommended the cyst on my scalp be removed by a general surgeon. The removal of this sebaceous cyst should have been a minor procedure and for a skilled dermatologist that would have been the case. Without doing any research, I blindly followed the doctor's advice and elected to have the cyst removed by a general surgeon who performed the procedure at a local hospital. Unfortunately, the surgeon who performed the procedure had little skill, and his area of expertise was obviously not cosmetic surgery. For reasons unknown, he deemed it necessary to shave a rather large area on the top of my head, and he proceeded to cut, pull, chop and tear away at the top of my head for what should have been a simple cyst removal. He closed the large incision with seven or eight stitches. I was left with an impressive scar at the very top of my head, suggesting the cyst removal was accomplished with human teeth rather than a scalpel. The unnecessary trauma to the area left the surgeon's signature where my hair never grew back.

Years later when I saw Dr. Kurnick for the poison ivy, I asked about three new cysts that were growing elsewhere on my scalp. These cysts were not painful or visible under the hair, but they were not paying rent and to have them homesteading on my head was persistently annoying. After he asked if I wanted to have them removed, I expressed apprehension by sharing the story of that previous disastrous experience with the general surgeon. Dr. Kurnick had a look at the top of my head then he made a wry face while shaking his head disapprovingly. After describing the simple procedure for removing these cysts, he said that he had successfully done "thousands of them." Dr. Kurnick then removed the three cysts from my scalp right there in his office, and I was pleasantly surprised when there was no shaving of my head. After anesthetizing each undesirable tenant with a needle and making the tiniest incision, he skillfully evicted each one, and then closed each incision with a single stitch, leaving no scars. After the procedure was completed, I sat there in a state of astonishment because his skills with a scalpel were nothing short of magical.

During the cleanup, Dr. Kurnick asked about my MS, and I brought up the subject of the clinical trial placebo effect. I explained my discovery of the success rates in the placebo groups, and how I was working on learning the placebo effect and mind control to fight the disease. I expected him to laugh but instead he brought up the Rogaine® (minoxidil) clinical trials, and he pointed out that 18 percent of the men in the placebo group of those trials actually started growing hair where they did not previously have it. As it turned out, Dr. Kurnick is a firm believer in the ability of the human mind to make changes to the body. I left his office elated about two things: I just had three cysts stealthily removed from my head, and this wizard had just given credence to my methods of fighting MS.

Chapter 17

People Who Accomplished the Impossible

Nando Parrado

> *"I turned myself into a survival machine. I didn't want to die."*

> **- Nando Parrado**

As it became increasingly clear that I was making a complete and remarkable recovery from MS, I often wondered why it was taking so long to write this book. Although I had been working on it sporadically for several years, an important part of the book was somehow missing and I was not even sure what it was. In the fall of 2012, the revelation of what was missing hit like a bolt from the blue. While walking on Spruce Street in front of the Kimmel Center, which is the Philadelphia Orchestra's home, I noticed a poster for the Weidner University Lecture Series for the 2012 – 2013 season. This poster escaped my attention on previous occasions, but this time a picture on the poster caught my eye   it was Nando Parrado. He was billed as the guest speaker for the series on April 15, 2013. Nando was one of the key people who unknowingly guided me during my recovery, and I never imagined the possibility of meeting him and personally expressing my gratitude. This was too good to be true because it was not just an opportunity to meet him, but it would happen on my home turf. Nando Parrado was giving a lecture at the Philadelphia Orchestra's home!

I read the book *Alive*, by Piers Paul Read, in 1977 during my first year at The Juilliard School in New York City. During my first two months at Juilliard, I temporarily resided with my grandmother in Queens, NY, before moving to a spacious 13 x 20 foot studio apartment on West 70th Street in Manhattan that had no kitchen. One day I wandered into a used book store on Broadway and there was a copy of the book *Alive*, which looked interesting, so I picked it up and started reading. Browsing used book stores was once a favorite pastime of mine, but this obsolete business model has unfortunately gone the way of 8-tracks, cassettes, rotary phones, black and white TV, and dial up internet. The book was a fascinating modern survival story. I purchased it, finished it rather quickly and reread it several times. Without any realization, I stored it away in my subconscious. *Alive* would remain dormant for twenty-two years until it would be called upon to help fight my own life-threatening survival situation.

On October 13, 1972, a Uruguayan rugby team was flying from Montevideo, Uruguay, to Santiago, Chile, for a rematch with a Chilean rugby team. The flight would cross the 150-mile wide Andes Mountain range, which is the largest mountain range in the world. The plane was a small twin propeller with a capacity of forty-five people plus two pilots and one member of the flight crew. After leaving Montevideo, bad weather in the Andes forced the plane to land east of the range in Mendoza, Argentina. Following a delay of several hours, the weather in the mountains improved and the pilot made the ill-fated decision to proceed west across the Andes. Not long into the flight, the plane encountered bad weather, and the pilot radioed air traffic control in Santiago that he was proceeding to turn north for the landing in Chile, which is on the western side of the mountain range. Suddenly, radio communication with the plane was lost and there was no further contact. The plane was reported lost and over the next few weeks extensive searches for the plane took place, but eventually they were called off due to the slim chances anyone could have survived a crash in the Andes Mountains during the winter. To make matters worse, the plane was white and there was little chance searchers would ever spot a white plane in the snow from high above the peaks. The snow in the mountains that winter was the heaviest snowfall in fifty years, making any chance for any survival even more dismal.

As it turned out, there was almost no visibility at the time of the crash, and for reasons that will remain unknown, the pilot brought the plane down for a landing in the middle of the mountain range. On the initial impact, the wings and the tail of the plane were sheared off but the plane miraculously landed on its belly. Amazingly, the fuselage continued a high-speed, 2,000-foot sliding descent down a snow-covered mountain without hitting any rocks. As the plane came to a stop in the snow, the abrupt deceleration caused many injuries and fatalities. Seat mountings broke loose, and people were thrown forward, including Nando, who went from row nine into the bulkhead, fracturing his skull in four places. Two of the survivors who happened to be medical students, immediately began seeing to the needs of the injured. When they examined Nando, his face was swollen, covered with blood, and he had no detectable pulse, so they determined he was dead. Nando was then placed in the cold along with the bodies of those who had perished, but that intense cold miraculously kept Nando's brain from swelling, thereby saving his life.

Surprisingly, Nando awoke from his coma three days later, and just four days after that he realized they were not going to be rescued. At that point, he knew their only chance of survival was to climb out and rescue themselves. Climbing out would be nearly impossible. The plane had come down in a giant bowl in the middle of the Andes that was surrounded by huge mountain peaks. It was winter, and the plane had come to rest on a glacier at an altitude of 11,500 feet. Heavy snowdrifts were ten feet deep in places, and the nighttime temperatures dropped to 30 and 40 degrees Fahrenheit below zero.

Seventy-two days after the plane went missing, all hope had been lost, but to the surprise of the world, two passengers on that flight, Nando Parrado and Roberto Canessa, showed up in a remote area high in the western foothills of the Andes. This truly remarkable modern survival story captured the hearts and imaginations of the world, and it became a source of inspiration for many, including me.

How did Nando survive a life-threatening situation when the rules said there would be no survival? He had no wilderness survival training, had never climbed mountains, had never even seen snow, and yet he survived in an inhospitable environment where it was considered impossible to survive.

Nando accurately fits the *U.S. Army Survival Guide* description of someone with no survival training or skills. Not only did he survive, but also he did it with energy to spare and in some ways made it look easy. In a life-threatening situation, he did not follow the accepted rules, but instead he followed his own rules. Where did he find such motivation in a situation that offered no hope? How could he have had such endless energy in an environment that offered only bitter cold and desolation? What enabled him to climb and trek thirty-seven and a half miles through one of the world's most difficult mountain ranges during a brutal winter with no gloves, boots, ice axe, ropes or a tent? What kept him going for seventy-two days with almost no food? Nando obviously has the ability to concentrate and focus his mind at a superhuman level for extended periods, but more important is his tenacity and perseverance to never give up. He is a rare individual with a mental ability to defy hunger, severe discomfort, and physical and emotional pain. I am convinced that if Nando Parrado were placed in the placebo group of a clinical trial, he would be one of the subjects who would inexplicably improve. One has to wonder if Nando ever read the *U.S. Army Survival Guide*, for he could very well have written much of it.

In early 2013, the weeks leading up to Nando's lecture were filled with anticipation, and I felt like an excited child eagerly awaiting delivery of his new toy. I told my wife Teresa to put the date on our calendar because this event would take precedence over everything else. During the lecture, Nando spoke with the aid of a slideshow that included numerous photos of everything from the 1972 crash site, to current photos of his family. He spoke for over one hour then answered written questions submitted by members of the audience. Normally, I tend to get bored and fall asleep during long speeches. This was different. I recall the deafening silence in the hall as everyone was entranced by Nando's telling of his story.

As he went into detail about his fight for survival on the mountain, my sudden understanding of what a powerfully guiding force he had been during my struggle brought tears to my eyes. Astonishingly, there were many similarities between his struggle for survival and my battle with MS. He described the despair, hopelessness and misery of his situation on the mountain, and I could relate with a feeling of complete hopelessness during my lowest point with MS. People think of hell as a place with fire and heat, but Nando described the hell he knows as a cold and desolate place where there is no escape. I know hell as a place where everything you previously took for granted is mercilessly stripped away. Hell is the place where MS sadistically laughs while one is helpless to fight back and is forced to watch the disease slowly steal everything that is precious.

Hearing Nando speak was fascinating because he was unexpectedly modest and humble. Nando said he was no hero and insisted he possesses no special talents or skills, but I disagree because he has an unbending spirit and that exceptional will to never give up. While listening to Nando, I realized just how methodical my game plan against MS had been. Not only had I devised an effective and thought-out strategy, but also I followed it with discipline and determination and I never looked back.

A professional mountain climbing team later retraced Nando's thirty-seven and a half mile trek in similar winter conditions, and the team leader said there was no way Nando could have completed the journey had he known the distance and extreme difficulties ahead. Those thirty-seven and a half miles were treacherously hard miles, and what makes the trek even more inconceivable is the fact that Nando should have been extremely weak from the lack of food and his weight loss of 90 pounds. When Nando and Roberto finally reached help in the foothills of the Andes, the Chilean Air Force pilot of the rescue helicopter said he would never be able to find the crash site from Nando's indicated location on a map of the Andes. With that being the case, Nando promptly boarded the rescue helicopter and successfully guided the pilot back to the crash site.

That admirable and unselfish act of heroism is one of the inspiring reasons I strive to help others with this book. In the lecture, Nando told of his small and achievable goals on his journey, and the completion of each goal kept him from losing hope. During my long fight with MS, I had no clue how difficult the entire process would be or how long it would take, but each goal was an achievable one. After reaching a goal, I immediately raised the bar to a new and higher goal, and remained focused until that next goal was reached.

The best part of Nando's lecture was meeting him afterward. Since the Kimmel Center is the home of the Philadelphia Orchestra and the musicians have access to most of the building, my wife Teresa and I went backstage at the conclusion of the lecture to wait for Nando outside of his dressing room. We had coats and a heavy camera bag, so I suggested placing these items on top of my backstage cello locker off stage right, as we had no idea how long the wait would be. After placing all of our paraphernalia on top of my locker, I heard Nando's voice about twenty feet away and realized he had unexpectedly exited stage right. We went over to talk to him, but he was busy discussing logistics with four people from GDA Speakers who had sponsored the lecture. Teresa and I waited patiently for a chance to speak with him. During our wait, Nando kept glancing at me out of the corner of his eye.

During a lull in the conversation, I stepped forward and introduced myself as a cellist in the Philadelphia Orchestra. I told him of my dream to one day meet him and thank him for being one of the key people who guided and helped me get my life back. Nando seemed quite interested as I explained my diagnosis with MS fourteen years earlier, my prospects of permanent disability and my refusal to accept it. The highlight of the meeting was when I told Nando that because he had accomplished the impossible, I was able to accomplish the impossible. Nando smiled, leaned forward and gave me a bear hug! It was a truly powerful moment in my life. As an incredible energy radiated from him, it suddenly became clear how I was able to achieve what I did by following his extraordinary example of exceptional human will.

There are events in our lives that seem to slow down time, and this was one of those moments. As I looked into Nando's eyes, much of the past fourteen years of my life began to play out in slow motion, and for the first time I was hit with the distinct feeling that I had actually cured myself of MS. Before that point, I was not sure if the MS was in remission or if I had a case of benign MS, but for the first time I somehow knew the disease was gone. Nando's survival story was my guidebook and roadmap, and I had followed it with determination and perseverance. I now fully understood my battle with MS was not a fight against an illness, but an actual fight for my survival. Like Nando, I battled against overwhelming odds and lived to tell about it. The hopelessness, the fight, and the victory, had made me a stronger person in every way.

Nando seemed moved by my story and graciously obliged for a photo op, so Teresa captured a great moment of the two of us, which is proudly kept as the wallpaper of my phone where it is viewed several times each day. Before we left Nando asked for a copy of the photo. I emailed it along with a letter, but I honestly never expected to hear back from this busy survival superstar. Much to my surprise, his sister Graciela replied a few days later. Not knowing anything about Graciela, I searched her name and stumbled upon the documentary, *I am Alive* from the History Channel. This video is an excellent portrayal of Nando's amazing story, as it includes extensive interviews with key people, including one with Graciela. I replied to Graciela expressing gratitude for taking the time to write, and said I would not bother her anymore, as she must have so much email to handle. Two days later Nando warmly replied to my email as my story obviously interested him.

I wrote this letter to Nando Parrado:

April 17, 2013

Dear Nando,

Meeting you on April 15, 2013 was a dream for many years as I always wanted the chance to thank you for your help with my struggle that began fourteen years ago. I first read the book *Alive* in 1977, and was fascinated by this modern survival story and your unwillingness to give up.

In August of 1999, I was incapacitated with a severe case of Multiple Sclerosis, my third vicious attack that year, with near total loss of eyesight and the use my hands. I could hardly walk and my future looked nonexistent. The doctor at Wills Eye Hospital in Philadelphia said, "I will write you a note for permanent disability," and the impact of those words was no doubt similar to what you must have felt when you reached the summit and saw nothing but an expanse of snowcapped mountains. At that moment I felt my life was over.

Luckily I made a rash decision then just as you did, which also saved my life. I told the doctor he could keep his note and that I would go back to playing cello in the Philadelphia Orchestra six weeks later when the new season started. He asked how I was going to do that, since he believed it would be impossible to do so. I did go back but seeing and playing the cello were nearly impossible, but like you I did not give up. I kept playing and never missed a day. Over the next three years I struggled, but kept conditioning my mind to heal the body and to stay positive. During that time I changed everything about my life including diet, exercise and mental discipline. My eyesight and playing have returned, and I have been totally asymptomatic for fourteen years now! For the past ten years I have been off all medication and am in better physical condition at age fifty-four than I was at twenty.

During my recovery I reread the books *Alive* and *Miracle in the Andes* many times to find the secrets of your determination. You were such an amazing inspiration to accomplish what is impossible, and without your help and example I don't believe I could have been successful. I have read books by people who have MS and manage with it, and books by people who have it and have succumbed, but I have never read one by someone who did the impossible by beating the disease outright. You are an entire chapter in the book I am working on and I will make sure you receive a copy when it is completed. I am hopeful this book will be the first of its kind and it will help others with their struggle, no matter what the challenge may be.

In your lecture on April 15, 2013, you said, "Life is not measured by the number of breaths we take, but by the moments that take our breath away."

Meeting you was indeed a moment that took my breath away. Thank you so much for all you have done to give me a second chance at life.

Always,

Bob Cafaro

Cellist, The Philadelphia Orchestra

This is Nando's touching reply:

April 18, 2013

Dear Bob...many thanks for your warm and extraordinary message. I am humbled at your efforts and resilience. If I had something to do in making you feel better and have a new life, it makes me feel very well and that in some way, what I accomplished has some other meanings, than having a beautiful family.

It would be a great honor to be part of your book and I sincerely hope that our paths will cross again soon.

You are the real true statement of courage and determination...not me..! You crossed over the highest peaks of life and we should learn from you too.

With a big and strong hug,   Nando

Nando's Decisions:

Nando made several key decisions during his ordeal, and had he guessed wrong on any one of them, he would not have survived to tell his remarkable story.

1. The flight was open seating. He decided to sit in row nine. Upon impact, the tail of the plane was ripped off. Everyone in row ten and back, perished.

2. Initially, Nando took a window seat in row nine, and his teammate Panchito Abal took the aisle seat. During the flight, Panchito asked if they could switch seats so he could have a better view of the mountains. Nando agreed and gave up the window seat. Upon impact, the wing was torn off the plane and the propeller cut through the fuselage below the window, killing Panchito.

3. Four days after awakening from his coma, Nando was certain they were not going to be rescued, so he decided to get out on his own.

4. The plane had come to rest in a gigantic bowl in the middle of the Andes Mountain Range. The survivors had no idea where they were. It took three days to climb the mountain to the west. During that climb, Nando anticipated standing on the summit and looking at lush green Chilean valleys and houses with chimneys. Instead, when he reached the top, he saw a continuous expanse of snow covered mountains as far as the eye could see. Having no illusions, Nando knew any choice offered only death, but he made the decision to continue hiking west until he died.

Miracle in the Andes

In 2006, I was so excited to have a copy of Nando's new book, *Miracle in the Andes* that I read it in one day. This book is straight from the source and it differs from the first book, *Alive*, which was written by Piers Paul Reed thirty-three years earlier. *Alive* is more of a factual account. It dwells on details, squabbles and disagreements among the survivors. Nando's book *Miracle in the Andes*, illustrates the hope and despair, but always portrays each of the survivors in a positive light. Human emotions are brought to life and Nando never utters a negative word about any of his teammates on the plane. At first, I thought it was a sugarcoated account of his ordeal, but as I read further, it became clear that the writing is a reflection of Nando's warm and positive outlook. His qualities of seeing everything from an optimistic vantage point are exactly what enabled him to survive the seventy-two days on the mountain and trek those thirty-seven and a half miles. His altruism is what enabled him to board the helicopter and immediately head back to the crash site to save the others. Nando's combination of determination and selflessness made it possible to put his hunger, cold and exhaustion aside, and remain focused on rescuing the others.

It was extremely helpful to have the knowledge of and admiration for those who did the impossible, but it was even more important to mentally put myself in their situations to understand how difficult and hopeless their struggles actually were. In the fictional novel *Lord of the Flies* by William Golding, a group of young boys is stranded on a tropical island with no adults present to maintain order. Since there is no discipline or societal structure, the situation quickly deteriorates and turns to savage mayhem. Although the book is fiction, it illustrates what can happen when there are no rules or order in a survival situation.

While this chapter is about Nando, the credit goes not only to him, but also to all those who survived that ordeal. From the moment after Nando's plane crashed in the Andes, the survivors immediately established a form of government in the fuselage, because only a strict and orderly society would enable the group to survive such inhospitable conditions for such an extended period. There was no prior group survival training for what they encountered and to expect complete discipline was not realistic, but they worked amazingly well as a unit, and their accomplishment as a group is nothing short of admirable. One major advantage for the survivors was their group training as a rugby team. When an athlete trains, a particular skill or play is repeatedly drilled; this is known as "task-specific repetition." With this, the athlete develops what is known as "instinct born of training." This enables one to accomplish difficult tasks at a subconscious level, even when one is nervous and under extreme pressure.

After the plane crashed, the fuselage was left with a giant hole where the tail had been torn off. Protection from the intense cold was the first priority so everyone who was able immediately built a wall out of luggage to seal the hole, in order to get through the first night on the mountain. This wise move proved invaluable, not just for the first night, but also for each of the following nights. During the subfreezing nights, the team huddled closely together to share body heat and conserve precious energy. They strictly rationed the small amount of food that was collected after the crash. After that, the only remaining source of food was the bodies of those who perished in the crash. Even with this gruesome prospect as their only chance of survival, organization and discipline were still followed when distributing the new food source. Extra care was taken to ensure the most nutritious body parts were provided to those who were chosen for the expeditions so they would have the adequate strength required.

One particular example of this structured society took place when a tube of toothpaste was stolen from the rations, and one person was suspected of the crime. Considering the food that was available, the taste of toothpaste was a needed treat for everyone. The group of survivors held a meeting and the person suspected of stealing the toothpaste was brought up on charges of theft. At this makeshift tribunal, the empty toothpaste tube was presented as evidence, and the culprit was found guilty of theft. He was subsequently sentenced to give up his rations of cigarettes for several days, and he agreed to accept the punishment.

Even though I was fighting MS on my own, I knew it was important to act like a team in every sense. The discipline of getting the mind and body to work together in team spirit was vital to success. Hydration, a strict diet, meditation, training of the mind and staying positive could all be viewed as individual players on a team. I was the coach, coordinating everything from the sidelines. I followed Nando's path and mentally placed myself in his position. If I went out on disability, I knew it would be the same as Nando remaining in the fuselage of the plane: waiting for a rescue that would never come. Nando was certain there would be no rescue just as I was certain no new miracle drug would come along to cure me of MS. The Avonex® injections I was taking only provided statistical odds of slowing down the progression of the disease and not reversing it. Therefore, I found the challenges and parallels that applied to my fight with MS. Nando survived the impossible; therefore, I would survive the impossible.

Comparisons with Nando Parrado

The initial impact of the crash was devastating. Nando's skull was fractured in four places and he was in a coma for three days.	My diagnosis of MS was different but just as traumatic. I lost the use of my hands and eyes, and was barely able to walk. I was not in a coma, but awake and lucid to see everything that had been stripped away. Even though I was not lying in the freezing cold at a high altitude, my situation appeared equally hopeless. I knew if I stayed there and accepted what MS had in store, it would be the end of my life. Just as Nando had done, I was determined to escape and claw my way out.
On the glacier, everyone was very weak due to the thin air and lack of food.	My third attack stripped away all my strength, even small walks were exhausting and they left me gasping for breath.
Following the plane crash, the survivors were hopeful and believed rescue was imminent.	For the first few months after my diagnosis, I was hopeful and believed a rescue from Western medicine with a miracle cure was just around the corner.
Nando stood alone. He was realistic about not being rescued. After four days on the mountain, he was certain there would be no rescue. At that moment, he realized their only chance of survival was to get out on their own.	Shortly after being released from the hospital in 1999, it became clear there would be no rescue by Western medicine. At that point, I knew being cured of this horrible disease was something only I could do.
During his long trek, Nando thought not about himself, but unselfishly about his father and his colleagues on the plane. This remarkable attitude enabled him to board the helicopter to return to the crash site, after his thirty-seven and a half mile trek.	During my recovery, I began focusing not on my own needs, but on volunteer projects, which enabled me to keep pushing forward without looking back.

Throughout history, there have been amazing stories of survival. Nando's ordeal is an extremely detailed modern-day account of survival against impossible odds. Historians have not yet had the opportunity to modify the story because all of the survivors are alive today. Resorting to cannibalism was sensationalized by the media, but the survivors of the plane crash had only death as an alternative. Their seventy-two days high on a glacier in the winter is not just a survival story, it is an account of the limitless potential of the human spirit that each one of us possesses. The story captures the human soul and imagination because of the incredible life force that gives us the ability to accomplish the impossible. When the plane crashed, Nando lost both his mother and his sister, whom he loved dearly. They were taken from him, but Nando's hope, dreams and spirit would not be taken. When I was at my low point with MS, everything was taken from me, including my eyesight, the use of my hands, and the ability to play the cello; but MS would not take my fighting spirit or my dreams. This is the lesson I learned from Nando, and it is a lesson we can all learn from this truly exceptional human being. Meeting Nando Parrado was truly a moment in life that took my breath away.

Nolan Ryan

"For me to be successful, I had to be aggressive." - **Nolan Ryan**

I am by no means a sports enthusiast, but I do have warm childhood memories of watching N.Y. Mets baseball games with my Great Uncle Phil. He was a kind person with a good soul, and an avid N.Y. Mets fan. While sitting back in his chair and puffing away on his beloved pipe, he often told stories of the great athletes. One of his favorites was the great fastball pitcher Nolan Ryan. I will never forget the one about the Amazing Mets' 1969 World Series, when they were in a jam against the Baltimore Orioles. The Orioles had the bases loaded with no outs. Rescue came from the bullpen when the Mets brought in the young Nolan Ryan. He took the mound and threw only eleven pitches to strike out the next three batters and end the inning.

Years later, when I got interested in the cello and became self-motivated, I was drawn to baseball pitching as a guide. The intricate mechanics and coordination required to throw a baseball at a major league level are similar to playing the cello. The connection may not be obvious to someone who never played the cello, but the skills of playing a musical instrument are inherently athletic. In sports and music, the common ground is timing of body movement. I tell my cello students that your fingers are the ten players of the team and you are the coach, so your job is getting those ten players to work together.

My next memory of Nolan Ryan was in 1977 when he pitched for the California Angels. This was a pitcher's duel between two of the best in the game, Ron Guidry of the N.Y. Yankees and Nolan Ryan. Both pitchers gave a masterful performance and the Angels bested the Yankees by the score of 1 – 0. Even though I watched this game on a small black and white television, it was fascinating to see the display of coordination by both pitchers. Ron Guidry was famous for his 95-mph slider, a pitch that dipped down as it approached the plate, and Nolan Ryan was famous for that 100-mph fastball. At that time, the Yankees were considered baseball's dominant team, and their lineup boasted some of the best power hitters in the league.

This was a game where both pitchers were amazing, but Nolan demonstrated particularly good form with his fastball traveling at speeds that had to be in the 100-mph range. That velocity combined with the intense spin applied to the ball, actually made the ball rise as it approached home plate. It is difficult enough to hit a baseball traveling at a speed of 100 mph, but to hit a ball at that velocity with unexpected upward motion is nothing short of impossible. Throughout the game the great Yankee batters were swinging at air, and they were unable to score a single run. It was a great experience to watch this game, and I had no idea it would one day be replayed in my head with a specific purpose in mind.

After graduating from The Juilliard School in 1980, my first job was teaching cello at the University of Virginia in Charlottesville, Virginia, from 1980 – 1983. During those three years, I resided in a single-family rental house on a cul-de-sac in a quiet family neighborhood. Directly across the street lived a family with a young boy, and each day the boy and his father pitched a baseball out on the street. Over the next three-years, I watched this boy develop solid pitching skills, and by the end of my tenure he was displaying good form and delivering the ball with some impressive velocity. Watching this on a regular basis instilled a desire to one day have a son and teach him how to pitch a baseball.

It wasn't until years later, during the beginning of my recovery that Nolan Ryan would become a major presence in my life. My young son Ryan joined Little League baseball and was recruited to pitch. This was my chance to live that experience of pitching with my son every day. I had the desire to help, but possessed little knowledge about pitching, therefore I made a trip to the local bookstore that yielded an unexpected discovery: *Nolan Ryan's Pitcher's Bible*. This book was exactly what I had been looking for but it would turn out to be much more.

Why is Nolan Ryan a chapter in a book about beating MS? Nolan Ryan is known as an amazing pitcher, but the reason for his inclusion in this book is his impossible accomplishment of staving off the aging process of the human body for twenty-five years. He pitched in the Major Leagues for twenty-seven seasons until he retired at the age of forty-six. His fastest pitch was 100.9 mph and he holds the record of 5,714 strikeouts. At age forty-four, he pitched his record seventh no hitter, and in that game the velocity of his pitches were clocked as high as 96 mph. That success did not come easily. Nolan paid the price by making all the necessary sacrifices that enabled him to achieve such results and longevity. All year round, his lifestyle, diet, exercise regimen and mental discipline were geared toward keeping his body in top physical condition for the next game.

We live in a society that is in a perpetual search of an elusive fountain of youth. We spend a great deal of time and money on products and elective surgeries that feed on that hope of regaining youth. Of course we all want to look and feel younger but we overlook the obvious answer that is right in front of us: lifestyle. Nolan Ryan certainly had good genetics, but genetics will take a person only so far. This is similar to a musician who relies only on raw talent. The truly great musicians are those who work the hardest and understand the limits of relying on talent alone. Nolan's book clearly spells out exactly what enabled him to be so good for such a long period. He earned the right to keep his body in his twenties while he was in his forties.

I began reading Nolan Ryan's book only to help my son, but the book had several missing pieces of the recovery puzzle that fell into place. Could Nolan Ryan's detailed account of staving off the aging process be effectively applied to staving off or even reversing an illness? So much can be learned from Nolan Ryan because he was constantly on the lookout for a better mousetrap. His intense thought process never ceased as he continually analyzed the timing and details of every movement when pitching. His trademark high leg lift wind up, the twist of his torso, and that precise moment of releasing the ball, were all given extensive analytical thought.

One unexpected and invaluable benefit from researching Nolan Ryan was the way it helped me reclaim and even exceed my previous level of cello playing. In 1999 when my brain's communication was cut off from the muscles, it was necessary to find new ways for the brain to communicate, so I began following Nolan Ryan's example of a tireless work ethic to take back what had been stolen from me. Nolan's quote, "To compete with guys half my age, I have to work twice as hard," became my own motto. I was competing with MS, a formidable opponent. Nolan was renowned for his four-hour daily workouts. For me four hours would not be enough; I decided to devote twenty-four hours a day, seven days a week to beating MS.

Nolan Ryan thought outside the box. Pitchers were not allowed to weight train back then. In his book, he credits weight training for his strength, endurance and longevity. Without the knowledge of his team, he had a Nautilus machine installed in his home. I had already been practicing yoga on a daily basis, so to emulate Nolan Ryan I bought a set of Olympic weights and a bench. I incorporated weightlifting into my daily exercise routine. A standard set of weights would have no doubt achieved the desired results, but the photos in Nolan's book picture him using a set of Olympic weights. It was vital to become Nolan Ryan in every possible sense, therefore only a set of Olympic weights would suffice.

As a cellist I was rightly concerned about longevity from the effects of wear and tear on my joints during the repetitive lifting of heavy weights, so I modified lifting to fit my own needs with a custom method of weightlifting. The notion of customizing weightlifting emerged from one paragraph in Nolan Ryan's book where he recommends using free weights instead of weight machines. He recommends foregoing machines that help support the weights and using free-weights instead. He also mentions increased muscular coordination that is achieved by balancing a set of dumbbells or a bar. Nolan Ryan believes free-weight exercises, performed with barbells or dumbbells are superior to weight machines because the body will support the weight instead of a machine. As a result, muscles built with this approach will be stronger, smarter and more useful than muscles developed with machines.

His philosophy struck me because it offered answers to my two biggest weaknesses caused by MS – physical strength and coordination. I took Nolan's system of weight training one step further and modified it to fighting MS instead of pitching a baseball. After some experimenting, I came up with a system of lift and hold rather than repetition, and for coordination, I use free weights exclusively. This system is what I call "MS Weightlifting." MS attacks the central nervous system and coordination; therefore Nolan's advice to use free weights became doubly important. I began lifting free weights on a daily basis and my strength and central nervous system slowly showed signs of improvement.

Lifting weights becomes even more beneficial as the body ages because weight-bearing exercise strengthens bone. Osteoporosis will be an unfortunate future reality for many people. Strengthening bone with weight-bearing exercise is an excellent way to reduce the chances of fracturing weakened bones later in life. In addition to my daily morning yoga and MS weightlifting, I also do chin-ups and handstands. When I adopted Nolan Ryan's lifestyle of exercise, diet and mind control, my only goal was to fight MS. The benefit that was unforeseen at the time was to have slowed my aging process by a remarkable degree. In addition to having beaten MS, I am in better physical condition at the age of fifty-seven than I was at age twenty.

One can only wonder what would have happened if Nolan Ryan had continued his disciplined regimen and lifestyle after he retired from pitching. I have little doubt he could have made the legendary fitness guru Jack LaLanne pale in comparison.

The mind control of Nolan Ryan:

During Nolan's warm-up in the bullpen prior to pitching his seventh no hitter, his pitching coach Tom House watched Nolan throw eighteen to twenty warm up pitches, and he predicted a disastrous performance on the pitching mound. House reported to Head Coach Bobby Valentine the bad news that Nolan "just doesn't have it tonight." After Nolan took the mound and retired the side in the first inning, he stood up and said to his teammates, "Boys, just get me one [run]. That's all I'm going to need tonight." He then retook the mound and went on to complete his legendary seventh no hitter.

It is important to look at the display of mental control Nolan had at that moment. He didn't just think he was in total control for the remainder of the game, he knew it. Nolan had no doubts about what was about to take place because he was fully in charge of both mind and body. There is a big difference between thinking something will happen and knowing it will happen. Fear and self-consciousness were nowhere to be found that night, as Nolan never lost his focus during the entire game. When the late Yogi Berra, a catcher famous for his witticisms, said, "90 percent of the game is half mental," it was funny but that quote contains a degree of seriousness. Baseball requires an extraordinary amount of physical conditioning, but it requires even more mental control and extreme powers of concentration. People often think of athletics as a skill of the body then the mind, but athletics is first a skill of the mind, then the body.

Fighting MS requires similar powers of mental control and concentration because this disease is an opponent with an enviable winning record. This is much more than a ballgame and the stakes are "winner takes all," so one must be willing to sacrifice anything and everything. It will take unprecedented sacrifice and discipline to completely change one's lifestyle. Self-motivation will be required as never before, and there must be a complete willingness to shun everything that could possibly reduce the chances of victory. This includes a diet void of processed food and drink, the elimination of alcohol, tobacco, recreational drugs, and all stimulants. We are all capable of beating MS, but MS patients should not just think they can beat it – they must *know* they can beat it. If there is any doubt, there is no doubt, and it is vital to be a total believer of what one is capable of accomplishing.

Shortly after his retirement from baseball, Nolan went on to become the owner of the Texas Rangers. After acquiring the team, a reporter asked him if he foresaw ownership of the team and Nolan replied: "No, I didn't think I would become owner of the Texas Rangers, but I never thought I'd pitch seven no-hitters either." This is yet one more example of the remarkable qualities of this driven person who refuses to sit back and live off the interest.

Comparisons with Nolan Ryan

Nolan Ryan knew if he relaxed during the off-season, time and his age would catch up with him and he would lose his magic.	I knew if I stopped playing the cello, I would never be able to play again. This was the main reason for going back to work at the earliest possible opportunity. Down time would have meant dead time.
Nolan Ryan devoted much of his life to his pitching, even in the off-season.	I devoted even more of my life to fighting my illness, because MS has no off-season.

When warming up for his 7th no hitter, things looked hopeless, but after the first inning Nolan knew the game was his.	After eight months with MS, things looked hopeless, but I trained the body and mind, and earned the right to know I would win.
Nolan Ryan said, "For me to be successful, I had to be aggressive."	For me to be successful in beating MS, the word aggressive had to take on an entirely new meaning.
To stay in shape in the off-season Nolan Ryan built a gym in his home.	Following his example, I bought an Olympic set of weights and worked with them daily.
After the first inning of his 7th no hitter, Nolan announced to his teammates he would need just one run. He did not *think* he would shut down the opposing team, he *knew* it.	When I made the decision to stop taking Avonex® in September of 2003, there was no doubt in my mind. I did not *think* I had beaten MS for good, I *knew* it.

Bobby Fischer (March 9, 1943 - January 17, 2008)

Who in their right mind would consider Bobby Fischer a guide for beating MS? He may have been a chess genius, but he was also a paranoid, antisocial, anti-Semitic misogynist. Looking beyond his many bizarre issues, Bobby Fischer was one of my guides. He accomplished the impossible in beating the Soviet state sponsored chess machine in 1972 when he won the World Chess Championship.

For much of the twentieth century, keeping the World Chess Championship in Soviet hands was a top priority for the Communist state. If a young child in the Soviet Union displayed an exceptional aptitude for chess, that child was indoctrinated into the chess system and the family was given special privileges in order to focus entirely on the child's development. This was not merely a game to the Soviet government, but a matter of national pride. Wresting the crown from Soviet hands eluded the rest of the world for decades, until Bobby Fischer's victory in 1972. Fischer was a self-taught kid from Brooklyn, New York, and his accomplishment places him up on a level with Nando Parrado and Nolan Ryan.

My older brother Billy taught me how to play chess as a child, but I never had much interest in the game until my first year at Juilliard when I went into

Coliseum Books, which was one of the largest bookstores in Manhattan. I was browsing through their extensive book selection and noticed an entire section on chess, so I purchased a book written in 1963 titled *The Complete Book of Chess*, by I.A. Horowitz and P.I. Rothenberg. I figured that learning the game would be a good brain exercise. An entire chapter of this book is devoted to the young Bobby Fischer, who was already seen as the great American hope for the elusive world title.

My chess lessons commenced when I replayed the thirteen-year-old Fischer's 1956 masterpiece, "The Game of the Century." This remarkable game was rightfully named because of its unprecedented depth, creativity and foresight. A game at this level by any Grandmaster would be amazing, but such a game from a thirteen-year-old is not of this world. In most chess books, the games are annotated by a chess Grandmaster to help understand the moves, but in this book, they were not. My knowledge of chess fundamentals was very limited, so most of the moves in this game made no sense. In need of some fundamental training on the game, I returned to Coliseum Books and bought two more books on chess. One was *Chess The Easy Way,* by the Grandmaster Reuben Fine, and the other was *My 60 Memorable Games*, by Bobby Fischer. Now that I was officially bitten by the chess bug, much of my time away from the cello was spent learning from Fischer's book.

The lessons that I learned from Fischer's games were invaluable. They were not just lessons in chess, they were lessons in life. The knowledge and insight attained from his games, thought process and particularly his annotations, would later become crucial tools when fighting MS.

An example from Fischer's book is game 58, where Fischer plays against Efim Geller, the Soviet Grandmaster who would later be Boris Spassky's assistant during the 1972 World Championship match against Fischer. In this game against Geller, Fischer has a winning position, but on the twentieth move, he makes a mistake and loses the game four moves later.

There is a moral of the story, which appears at the end of the game: "It is not enough to be a good player. You must also play well." This applies not only to chess, but it also applies to cello playing and many aspects of life as well. People should never fall into complacency, and throughout life, they should take pride in everything they do. When it came to fighting MS, this meant never letting my guard down, even for one minute.

One other example is game number 9 against a relatively unknown Swiss Grandmaster, Edgar Walther. By move 36 Fischer is in a completely lost position and ready to resign, but Walther makes one subtle mistake. Fischer cleverly takes advantage of the error and winds up drawing the lost game. The moral of the story in this game is: "The good player is always lucky." The lesson learned here has little to do with luck, but it is about never giving up, no matter how hopeless a situation may seem. During my struggle with MS, it would be an understatement to say things looked hopeless, but I never gave up and in the end, the reward was a win and not a draw.

One of my favorite examples in Fischer's book is his intense rivalry with Mikail Tal, another Russian who went on to become the world champion. At their meeting in a 1959 tournament, the sixteen-year-old Fischer played four games against Tal and lost all four games. After winning the tournament, a chess fan asked Tal for an autograph, and he obliged by signing Fischer's name. Tal then explained, "I have beaten Bobby so often that it gives me the right to sign for him." Fischer did not get discouraged or give up, but instead he focused and worked even harder. At their next meeting in 1960 which is game 23 in Fischer's book, the improved Fischer played Tal to a draw in a hard fought game that is incredibly complex, and on the fifteenth move in this game, Fischer uncharacteristically thought for almost one hour. Fischer continued to work and improve, and one year later (game 32), he finally beat Tal for the first time. In Fischer's book, he clearly illustrates this rivalry was about much more than chess. It was about being overwhelmed by a superior opponent and losing a battle with humiliating defeat, then regrouping, rebuilding, and returning stronger to win the war.

Bobby Fischer sacrificed anything and everything to win chess games. His preparation was unparalleled and he had superhuman powers of concentration. He always thought outside the box and constantly studied in search of finding better ways to win at the chessboard. At the chessboard Bobby Fischer was proactive, not reactive, and he thought further ahead than his opponents did. Fischer was such a dominating force in chess because he worked harder and worked smarter than everyone else, and when he played chess nothing else in the world existed. His mind was totally focused; to him chess was not a game, but a fight for his life. He was determined not to lose. When he did lose a game, he spent a great deal of time analyzing exactly what had gone wrong to ensure it would never be repeated.

Bobby Fischer paid a heavy price for his unique ability to withdraw into the chessboard. As a young teenager, he became intolerant and impatient with everyone and everything outside of his chess world. He dropped out of high school at the age of sixteen, and his social skills were nonexistent as he had little use for friends or any social life. Perhaps Fischer's downfall was his exclusive focus on a single material goal, and that goal was to win the Chess World Championship. After achieving that goal in 1972, Fischer dropped off the face of the earth and went into seclusion. Perhaps he achieved his material goal and he no longer saw a reason to continue.

Regardless of his social shortcomings, Bobby Fischer offers much to model after when it comes to battling MS. I put myself in his position because chess was not a game to Fischer, but it was the ultimate struggle in many respects. He valued chess above all else and his self-respect was measured by success at the chessboard. I became Bobby Fischer, the self-taught kid who took on the Soviet establishment and its culture, and won. I was the underdog who would rise from the ashes to beat an established disease that proudly displayed an unbeatable record. There would be definite social costs with this undertaking, but the prospect of an unfavorable outcome forced a willingness to sacrifice whatever was necessary to win. *My 60 Memorable Games* offers incredible insight into the thought process of his genius mind and how he was able to outthink and outsmart his opponents. Bobby Fischer was one of the very best prepared players of his day, and his extensive preparation gave him detailed knowledge of openings, middle games and endings of so many previously played games. While playing chess or immersing himself in preparation for his games, nothing else existed in Fischer's world, and the intensity of his concentration was unparalleled.

Comparisons with Bobby Fischer

Chess was not just a game to Fischer. It was a fight to the death.	MS was not just a disease. It was a fight for my life.
Fischer devoted his entire life to winning chess games.	From the time I was released from the hospital, I devoted my entire life to beating MS.
Chess took precedence over everything for Fischer, including his social life.	Fighting MS was the focus of my life and everything else was secondary.

During his 1959 meeting with Tal, Fischer was no match but he persevered with determination, and eventually earned the ability to overtake Tal.	During my first eight months with MS, I was pitted against a completely overwhelming opponent. Over the next two years, I devoted everything to successfully winning any future meetings.
Fischer had no friends and had little patience for people in general.	Luckily, this is where my comparisons with Bobby Fischer end.

Jascha Heifetz (February 2, 1901 - December 10, 1987)

"If you think I'm tough on you, remember, I'm twice as tough on myself."

- Jascha Heifetz

Jascha Heifetz was a major source of inspiration. I never had the chance to hear him play live, but I was fortunate to have studied cello with Channing Robbins, my cello teacher at Juilliard from 1976 – 1978. Channing frequently referred to Heifetz as "a God on the violin," and during my lessons, he was more than willing to share many firsthand stories and experiences. At times those cello lessons were motivational speeches, and his many stories stay with me as if I heard them yesterday.

One of my favorite stories is one that took place late in Heifetz's career when he phoned his colleague and friend, the great cellist Gregor Piatigorsky. Piatigorsky was teaching when Heifetz called and there were several students were present in the room; however, Heifetz insisted that he needed to talk to him right away about something very important! The urgent matter was that Heifetz had found a new way to warm up on the violin and he was excited to share the news of his discovery. As the story continued, Piatigorsky relayed the news to his students who were present while laughing about the matter. I was not laughing when I heard this, because it clearly illustrates why Heifetz belongs on this list of people who accomplished the impossible.

Perhaps the most important firsthand story from Channing Robbins was from the six years he played cello in the Cleveland Orchestra. Every season, Heifetz appeared with the orchestra as guest soloist, and each time he hibernated in his Green Room for two full hours before he took the stage. During each two-hour hiatus, he warmed up in a manner that only Heifetz could. It was possible to hear outside Heifetz's room, so Channing set up a folding chair outside the door, listened, and learned from the master.

Heifetz's routine began with some warm-up exercises to get his fingers ready, and then the serious work began. He began with the first difficult passage in the concerto he was about to play, first at a very slow tempo, then repeating it faster and faster until he brought it up to tempo. Things did not stop there. The passage was drilled yet faster and faster to the point it was way past tempo or "until it was a mess," as Channing said. This discipline was repeated with each passage in the concerto for the full two hours right up until the time he went out onstage, and then Heifetz performed at a breathtaking level of perfection. To play an instrument at Heifetz's level requires extraordinary organizational skill and discipline, and his intense focus during his warm up is a perfect illustration of what it takes to excel.

At the end of my second year at Juilliard, I attended a summer music festival in Vancouver, B.C., where I met a fabulous violinist named Jackie Brand. At that time, she was a student of Heifetz, and the master's famous work ethic had obviously been ingrained in her. We had a conversation about Heifetz and I told her how much I had learned from him. Jackie said if I wrote and told him exactly that, he would write back. Unfortunately, I never wrote to him and that is one of my many mistakes in my life that will always be regretted.

There are violinists who have played at Heifetz's level for a period, but not for sixty years! From his early teens until the time he stopped playing in 1972, Heifetz played at a level that was not human. Channing always said he was a God on the violin, and the senior members of the Philadelphia Orchestra who were fortunate enough to have heard him play live agree wholeheartedly. In the booklet included with Heifetz's *The Complete Album Collection*, there is an anecdote that took place when Heifetz was auditioning pianists. In 1944 the pianist Milton Kaye auditioned to be his accompanist and Heifetz began lecturing him, asking if he was ready for the discipline and sacrifices it takes to be an artist. Kaye was speechless because he had only come for an audition. Heifetz continued, "Remember. If you think I'm tough on you, remember, I'm *twice* as tough on myself."

Heifetz studied with the legendary violin teacher Leopold Auer, who had many students who went on to become great solo violinists. Auer's book, *Violin Playing as I Teach It*, is one of the books kept on display in my studio, and my favorite part is the chapter on tone production. He states that a violin tone is not produced by simply drawing the bow across the string, but it goes much further than mechanical sound production. "The violinist must be willing to sacrifice his entire soul and all he is capable of to accomplish this." When it comes to beating MS, there could be no better description of what is needed.

From my lowest point after my third attack, the work of relearning everything about playing the cello began from step one, so I started with open strings just trying to relearn how to make a good tone by drawing the bow. Analyzing every movement, I discovered subtle imperfections in the way I had previously used the bow. However, the left hand was a different story. Even though both my arms were still under the brain's command, the fingers were not following orders. For help I resorted to a video titled *Heifetz*, a black and white film from the early 1950s. In this film, Heifetz is shown practicing scales, but more important is his demonstration of finger exercises. I slowly began applying those exact same exercises to the cello several times each day, and over a period of time the control and dexterity of my fingers gradually began to improve and return.

If I were granted one wish in my life, it would be to see Heifetz perform live. Unfortunately his last recital took place in October 1972, several years before I became seriously interested in the cello. Heifetz raised the level of string playing to an entirely new standard and his example will always be admired. Not only did he leave a recording legacy that will never be equaled, he left the entire world of music in awe. After attending a concert by the young Heifetz, George Bernard Shaw wrote him a letter that said: "If you provoke a jealous God by playing with such superhuman perfection, you will die young. I earnestly advise you to play something badly every night before going to bed, instead of saying your prayers. No mortal should presume to play so faultlessly."

Comparisons with Jascha Heifetz

When I first heard ten-year-old Sarah Chang play the violin, it was so amazing that I told the Philadelphia Orchestra's former principal violist Joe DePasquale, she was like a young Heifetz. Joe immediately shot back, "You don't compare anybody to that guy, EVER!" In light of that statement, there can be no attempt at comparing myself to Jascha Heifetz. Keep in mind

Joseph DePasquale was a truly great violist, and he made several recordings with Heifetz, which can be found in *The Heifetz Collection.*

Lance Armstrong – The Good, the Bad and the Ugly

Many people were kind enough to have provided invaluable input and guidance in the preparation of this book, and most felt very strongly that Lance Armstrong should not be included. The reason he is included is that he was a vital piece of the puzzle in my recovery.

After years of consistently denying using banned performance-enhancing drugs to win races, Lance was finally forced to come clean and admit to doping. What made matters worse was the deplorable way he treated people and how he destroyed the careers of people who accused him of banned substance use. Rather than focus on the drugs that enabled his impossible accomplishment of winning the Tour de France an unprecedented seven times, it is more important to look at his accomplishment of beating an illness that should have killed him. Lance Armstrong was victorious over cancer that would have been fatal in most cases, then he resumed a career as a competitor in one of the world's most demanding athletic events. His book, *It's Not About the Bike - My Journey Back to Life,* was crucially helpful in my battle because I could relate to the hopelessness of his situation.

When Lance Armstrong was diagnosed with testicular cancer, he was a top cycling contender and a member of the French cycling team Cofidis. When the team learned of his diagnosis he was promptly dropped as a member, and it appeared his life was over. Lance's testicular cancer metastasized aggressively and rapidly spread into his lungs and brain. His cancerous testicle was surgically removed, he endured high levels of chemo to combat the lung cancer, and he underwent brain surgery to remove the cancer from his brain. His doctors told him he was facing a fifty percent chance of survival, but privately they confided he had only a twenty percent chance of survival. They also predicted he would never ride a bicycle after the brain surgery because his sense of balance would be permanently impaired. To survive advanced cancer is impressive and to make a complete recovery is remarkable. To survive the cancer, make a total recovery, then resume a career as a serious competitor in the world's most difficult athletic event, is a superhuman feat. Lance Armstrong's use of illegal and unethical drugs may have ended his career in disgrace, but he did not use illegal or unethical drugs to win his battle with cancer.

It is important to understand that Lance Armstrong was willing to do anything and everything to win not only cycling races, but to win at everything in his life – including the fight for his life. Even before knowing anything about his use of banned substances to dominate the sport of cycling, I had a feeling that cohabitating with Lance Armstrong could be a challenging endeavor. His personality is so strong and domineering that it might not take long for his partner to head for the exit. The qualities that brought him down are the same qualities that enabled him to beat a disease that is not as strong or domineering as he is. Lance Armstrong fully understood that his cancer was an opponent that did not play by the rules, so he did not limit himself to playing by the rules. He understood the importance of fighting cancer in the mind and he did so very effectively.

Similarly, if one plays by an existing and accepted set of rules when fighting MS, it is the equivalent of bringing a knife to a gunfight. Lance Armstrong may have dominated the Tour de France by playing outside of the rules, but he also beat cancer by playing outside of the rules. When faced with MS and permanent disability, I emulated Lance Armstrong and did not follow the accepted set of rules. I refused to accept the standard MS prognosis, so I wrote my own rules and followed those new rules with discipline. Cancer was not just an illness to Lance Armstrong, it was yet another competition and he would cross the finish line first. Winning is in his blood, and his "take no prisoners" attitude toward people and life is what enabled him to emerge victorious against cancer. Lance Armstrong was not afraid of cancer, and when the dust settled it was clear, the cancer was afraid of him. This is the same attitude I adopted when battling MS. Lance Armstrong cheated to win cycling races, but he also cheated to beat a life-threatening illness. Very few people will ever compete in cycling races but most people will compete against a life-threatening illness at some point their lifetime. This is where Lance Armstrong will always remain a role model.

Lance Armstrong's downfall is a tragedy, but it is even more tragic for the people who will never have him as a guide and source of inspiration when battling life-threatening illnesses. I was fortunate to have him as a guide when battling MS, and I will always be thankful for his inspiration. Had I fully emulated Lance Armstrong, I would have used performance-enhancing drugs for my Principal Cello auditions. Had I chosen this route, I might have won one of them. This is not a joke because some musicians actually take beta blockers (Inderal is a brand name) to control nerves during auditions, and I can say from experience that high-level auditions are indeed a true test of nerves.

Comparisons with Lance Armstrong

When diagnosed with cancer, Lance Armstrong's successful career was derailed and it seemed like the end.	Six months after my diagnosis with MS, my career was derailed and the end seemed even nearer. Cancer is far more curable than MS.
Lance Armstrong said: "Cancer picked the wrong person."	I followed in Armstrong's steps and said: "MS picked the wrong person."
During his recovery, Lance got back on the bike and set his goal for the Tour de France.	During my recovery I got back on the cello. Wanting to come back from the abyss and win a major race, I took principal cello auditions. For a 41-year-old cellist, these were the closest things to the Tour de France.
Armstrong used performance enhancing drugs to win races.	Luckily, this is where my comparisons with Lance Armstrong end.

Roger Bannister and the Four-Minute Mile

May 6th is a special date in my life for two reasons. On that date in 1985 I won the Philadelphia Orchestra audition and on the same date in 1954 a twenty-five-year-old British medical student named Roger Bannister made history by breaking the four-minute mile barrier. Running one mile (1,760 yards, or 1,609 meters) in less than four minutes was considered impossible until Roger Bannister showed the world otherwise. Before that time doctors and athletes said such a feat was beyond the limits of the human body, but once Bannister broke the barrier his record was quickly eclipsed and today it has been bested by almost seventeen seconds. While the sub-four-minute mile is still a worthy feat, it has now been accomplished even by students at the high school level. Anyone interested in the subject of MS may find it ironic that after breaking the barrier, Roger Bannister went on to finish medical school and became a neurologist. When a person believes something is impossible, it cannot be done, but when a person sees that something is possible, it is an achievable goal. There was a time when science said the world was flat, but it would be difficult to find anyone defending that argument today.

I refused to accept a future on permanent disability, so in my mind curing myself of MS became an achievable goal. There were no illusions about the difficulties ahead, but I was determined to find the elusive Achilles heel of this disease and was willing to spend my life doing so. If neurologists saw repeated cases of MS patients who were cured, MS would be redefined as a curable illness. Dr. Markowitz said, "You did the impossible" because he had apparently never seen someone with such a severe case of MS make a complete recovery and show no signs of the disease. Dr. Sergott seemed equally surprised upon seeing me for the first time after our "permanent disability" chat, fourteen years earlier. Several doctors have said that I must have been misdiagnosed because beating MS is impossible, but if that were the case it would mean five highly respected neurologists and one top neuro-ophthalmologist all erred in their diagnoses.

I am convinced MS is in many cases curable, and if I believed otherwise it would mean a life on permanent disability and this book would have never been written. Since I have broken the ice and have run the sub-four-minute MS mile, my goal is to help others accomplish the same and redefine MS as a curable disease.

Comparisons with Roger Bannister

> We both got busy and ran like hell!

What do these people who have accomplished the impossible have in common? They all have extreme powers of concentration and an ability to focus intensively. Even more important than any natural ability is an extraordinary level of self-motivation possessed by every one of them. Each person who served as my inspirational guide possessed a common trait of being extremely passionate about their goals, and their desire and discipline to achieve those goals. To beat a disease such as MS, it will not just take lifestyle changes and discipline, it will take intense passion. This is not a battle one can fight with fear. One must fight with the excitement of knowing they will win.

There is no rulebook for beating MS, so to emerge victorious one must be constantly on the lookout for signs and signals from the body offering better ideas and methods. To successfully beat MS, one must understand how and why people are able to accomplish things that are considered impossible. To accomplish the impossible it is necessary to stay hungry. In an interview, Jascha Heifetz said we live in a world with too many comforts and to do well we actually have to deny ourselves a few things. He said discipline is a necessity, even for enjoying life. A combination of passion, devotion, intensity, discipline and self-motivation is what it takes to do the impossible, and this is what it will take to beat MS.

Chapter 18

Cycling to the Train Station

I earned some early confidence from research, from studying people who accomplished the impossible, from gradual improvement of eyesight, and from successfully balancing on two wheels of a bicycle. The time had come for another challenge, so I decided to resume cycling the 3.5 miles to the train station when the orchestra's 1999 – 2000 season began. Weakness and frailty definitely had the upper hand at that point, so training for the regular commute began with seven mile round trip practice runs. The route to the train station includes one hill that was never a challenge, but after getting out of the hospital and having no strength, this hill felt like Mt. Everest. On my first dry run, I struggled and somehow summited the hill, but once there I dismounted and struggled to catch my breath. After several weeks of practice runs my strength markedly increased, so when the orchestra season began I regularly biked to the train station and even started carrying my full size Dahon folding mountain bike up the stairs to the platform. The stairway up to the elevated train platform is forty-five steps, and with a 30 lb. bike, it is a demanding workout by itself.

For the first few months after my third attack the rides to the station elevated my pulse and cardiovascular system to the point where both optic nerves experienced serious inflammation, exacerbating my already challenged vision. To counter the optic nerve inflammation I practiced twenty minutes of deep breathing on the train ride, which enabled my pulse, respiration and vision to return to what was then the new normal. For much of that season I remember standing on the elevated train platform and not being able to read the large white corporate logo sign on the nearby red brick office building. Reading that sign before the days of MS was easy and never got any attention, but now it was difficult to make out the easily read large bold letters.

As my days of bike commuting progressed, I became obsessed with cycling to all the concerts and rehearsals, even in the pouring rain. I bought a bright colored rain suit for the wet rides and picked up a set of powerful lights for the nighttime rides, which effectively prevented a case of road kill. Many of the Philadelphia Orchestra concert goers who regularly saw me on the train at night with the bike and in all kinds of weather, likely assumed I was marching to the beat of a different drummer. They probably thought I lost my driver's license for drunk driving, but they had no idea of what I was really dealing with. Reaching for that higher goal and refusing to give in to any MS-imposed restrictions was one of the best decisions made during my recovery.

Chapter 19

The 1999 – 2000 Philadelphia Orchestra Season

Rejoining the orchestra in September 1999 after the third attack was a serious physical and emotional challenge, but the anxiety leading up to it was far worse. Three colleagues from the orchestra visited me in the hospital and one of them, Derek Barnes along with his wife Meichen, actually brought me there to be admitted. That meant word in the orchestra that I had MS was officially out and there would be no more hiding behind any fictitious misdiagnosis or attempting to talk my way out of it.

Every three years the Philadelphia Orchestra Association and the musicians of the orchestra come to terms on a new collective bargaining agreement. This just happened to be the time when the previous contract expired and the new one commenced. On Monday September 20, 1999, the orchestra musicians gathered in the hotel across the street from the Academy of Music to vote on a new three-year contract that had been tentatively approved by the musician's negotiating committee. The prospect of showing up at this meeting was terrifying beyond belief because everyone in the orchestra would now know I had MS, and there would be no director of public relations to act as my spokesperson.

Barely able to see and somehow concealing my difficulty walking, I proceeded into the meeting room hiding behind a forced smile, prepared for the worst. The meeting was already in progress, and several colleagues who noticed my presence looked at me wide-eyed with surprise. There was a sudden pause when the musician who had the floor and was speaking from the microphone called attention to my return. After a warm announcement welcoming my return, the musicians gave a big round of applause. It was emotionally touching to have been greeted with open arms. Somehow, I had expected to be shunned by the group because of my dreaded illness. One memory of that day that stood out was when a violinist who seemed surprised to see me up and about said, "Wow, I heard really bad things about what happened to you." I told him, "Whatever you heard is not true. It's ten times worse!"

At the conclusion of the orchestra meeting, I went to the voting table and was handed a ballot, but was unable to read what I was voting on. Having no idea what was in the proposed contract, I checked the box next to the big NO and headed home, wishing with all my heart that the orchestra would go on strike because I had no idea how I was going to play. Later that day it was announced on the local news station that the contract had been ratified, and that meant the first rehearsal of the Philadelphia Orchestra's 1999 – 2000 season would begin at 10:30 AM the next morning.

The Threat Is Stronger Than the Execution

There was good reason to dread that first rehearsal, because it was utterly impossible to see the music or play the cello. Before the start of the rehearsal, I went to the orchestra library to speak privately with the librarian Nancy Bradburd, and I asked if there was a way she could enlarge a set of cello parts for me. Like the sweetheart she is, Nancy made up personalized oversized cello parts, and with the giant music, I sat in the back of the cello section on a stand by myself. When the rehearsal started, it was harrowing because both hands were useless, and my eyes were vacillating between hopeless and terrible. There were times during those first few weeks the optic neuritis was so bad and the optic nerves so raw, it was literally not possible to see there was actually music on the stand. For much of the first few months of the 1999 – 2000 season I mimed it, hoping the cellists, violists and bassists around me would be too busy playing their own parts to notice how badly I was doing. I followed the movements of the cellists in front of me and managed to keep my bow moving in the right direction most of the time. The MS did hit my hands hard but it luckily spared my arms, so I was able to keep the left arm vibrating and in the same general vicinity on the fingerboard of the cello as the others.

This continued for several months, but thankfully there were subtle improvements in both the eyes and the hands. Admittedly there were many concerts during the first part of that season when I sat there sweating, hoping people in the audience would not notice the freeloading anchor in the back of the cello section. During some of those concerts, I felt like the inspiration for the song *"Fakin' It"* by Simon and Garfunkel, but I persevered, never missed a day and stood up with a forced smile during the applause at the end of each concert. My contributions to the orchestra that season were admittedly less than exemplary, but drawing a line in the sand and going back to work turned out to be an invaluable physical and psychological advantage in my battle against MS. I was barely able to see the music or play the cello, but nothing stopped me or slowed me down for one minute.

The NFL Films Recording Session

Another harrowing experience was my first recording session with NFL Films in Mt. Laurel, NJ. It was October 1999 and William (Bill) Stokking, the Philadelphia Orchestra's former principal cellist and contractor for these recordings, asked me to play one of the sessions. It had only been one month since I rejoined the orchestra, and with both hands still useless and my eyesight doing little to guide me, I expressed serious reservations to Bill about being able to play a recording session. Bill always seemed to know what was best for me, so he refused to take no for an answer and insisted I play the session while assuring me everything would be fine. At the recording session the music was thankfully not difficult, but just sustaining long whole notes was challenging because holding the bow steady was still proving elusive. I somehow managed to get through the session without attracting too much attention, but I had little doubt it would be the last time I would ever be asked to play for the NFL Films recording sessions. I must have been a seriously good faker because I was asked to play all the following NFL Films recording sessions.

Carnegie Hall

How do you get to Carnegie Hall? Don't drive there.

My single worst memory from the 1999 – 2000 Philadelphia Orchestra Season was the orchestra's performance at Carnegie Hall on January 24, 2000. The renowned Simon Rattle was guest conductor for the subscription week, and the single work on the program was *Gurreleider* by Arnold

119

Schoenberg. This is a major twentieth century work for chorus and orchestra, and the cello part is horrendously difficult. To further compound the challenges of playing this work, the parts were sloppily prepared by a copyist whose handwriting suggested he held his pen with two hands. Orchestra musicians are accustomed to having neatly printed parts for good reason; therefore, when hand-copied music is on the music stand, it always provides a legibility challenge.

For reasons that will forever remain mysterious and unexplained, I drove the 100 miles from my home in Cherry Hill, NJ to Manhattan that day and parked the car in a free space on West 74th Street, four blocks from my previous New York City residence. While living in Manhattan, I kept a car on the street for over two years. In the process, I became well versed with all of the New York City parking tricks and secrets. Free parking is my modus operandi because Dad taught me the value and immense satisfaction of finding free parking in Manhattan. This had nothing to do with an ability to afford parking in a paid lot; it was about the thrill of the hunt. Street parking in Manhattan provides an opportunity for a person's primal being to thrive in a modern setting because it is an urban combination of both hunting and natural selection.

My vision at this time had improved over my low point five months earlier, but it was still anything but satisfactory. It was now January, 2000 and I was eager to make strides in my recovery and continually raise the bar. This was the first long solo drive I had done, and driving to New York City in that condition was stupid and suicidal. It should never have been attempted. After a surprisingly successful two-hour drive to Manhattan with no accidents and finding a free parking space, I took the subway from the nearby West 72nd Street stop downtown to West 30th Street for a follow-up appointment with the alternative medicine specialist, Dr. Ronald Hoffman. Following the appointment, I took the subway uptown to West 59th Street for the Philadelphia Orchestra's afternoon rehearsal at Carnegie Hall on West 57th Street. At the conclusion of the rehearsal, I walked nineteen blocks north to the car on West 74th Street. That long walk was the dumbest possible move because walking that distance in my condition was still as physically demanding as running the New York City Marathon. My physical state had improved over the last 5 months, but it was nowhere close to normal. Commuting to work by bike on a regular basis had built my endurance, so I incorrectly assumed my body could easily handle a walk of 1 ½ miles. As it turned out, my body was in no condition to handle what turned out to be a strenuous cardiovascular workout.

Arriving at the car barely able to breathe and ready to collapse, I was almost blind from an elevated pulse and severely inflamed optic nerves. At this point, there was no twenty-minute rest period for deep breathing to calm my optic nerves. The tight schedule mandated hustling back to 57th Street by 6:45 pm, to wait in the car for a free 7:00 pm parking space. In retrospect, driving the car with such impaired eyesight was stupid and outright dangerous.

Because it was January in New York City, it was now dark outside and the nineteen-block drive down Broadway to 57th Street was a nightmare as I was unable to see if the traffic lights were red or green. Cars around me were barely visible and it was nearly impossible to see if there were any pedestrians in front of the car. While driving down Broadway at little more than walking speed, I kept my head out the window in an attempt to see where I was going. New York City drivers are known for their inherent courteousness and patience, so it was comforting when motorists extended their greetings by blowing their horns and waving with one finger. I literally could not see where I was going, but several kind pedestrians graciously helped me with their location by shouting names of orifices and feminine hygiene products.

By some miracle, I arrived at a free 7:00 pm parking space on 57th Street outside Carnegie Hall without hitting any cars or pedestrians, but the real challenge was yet to come. The Philadelphia Orchestra's Carnegie Hall performance of Schoenberg's *Gurreleider* would begin in one hour. This massive work utilizes sixteen cellos and the crowded stage eliminated any possibility of sitting alone on the last stand with my oversized easy-reader music. During the concert, I sat on the last stand with Glenn Fischbach, a young cellist and recent graduate of the Curtis Institute of Music. It was Glenn's first time playing as a substitute with the Philadelphia Orchestra, and I felt it was better to sit with him rather than call in sick. Had I done so, the MS would have gotten the upper hand and had its way with me.

During the entire performance, the optic nerves were severely inflamed from that nineteen-block walk, and it never let up. Not only was it impossible to see the notes of the cello part, I could not even see there was music on the music stand. I could make out Simon Rattle was conducting but deciphering his movements was impossible. That concert was one of the most unpleasant musical experiences of my life. For the entire performance, I was reduced to synchronizing my movements with those of the cellists around me while my bow moved silently across the strings. It is therefore my mark of distinction to have performed at Carnegie Hall - as a mime - with one of the world's greatest orchestras.

When string players in a symphony orchestra share a stand, they depend upon each other for everything from the bowings to the entrances after counting measures of rest. A high level of teamwork takes place when sharing a stand, and if one is not doing what is expected there is no hiding it from a stand partner. Throughout that concert I was terrified by the only possible thought that could have been going through my young stand partner's head: "Dead wood at such an early age!"

Chapter 20

Alternative Medicine - Dr. Ronald Hoffman

Mary Ann Mumm, a good friend and a violinist with a passion for healthy living, recommended seeing Dr. Ronald Hoffman, a medical doctor in New York City who specializes in alternative medicine and holistic healing. Dr. Hoffman is a celebrity in the world of alternative medicine and since 1988, he is well known as host of the radio show "Intelligent Medicine" which is the longest-running physician-hosted health program on the air.

The cost of seeing this designer alternative medicine doctor was not covered by insurance. It would be a major expense, but at that point, I was willing to try anything. I phoned the Hoffman Center and they were able to accommodate my schedule with an appointment the morning of Tuesday October 19, 1999, the same day of the Philadelphia Orchestra's first Carnegie Hall concert of the 1999 – 2000 season. In 1999, the Hoffman Center was located on 40 East 30th Street between Madison Avenue and Park Avenue. It was six blocks from the subway stop on West 28th Street, which under normal circumstances would have been an easy walk. During my days as a Juilliard student and later as a cellist with the Metropolitan Opera Orchestra, I walked everywhere in Manhattan, but that was a time of perfect health.

When saddled with an advanced case of MS, walking time should be estimated by factoring current and not past health conditions. The six-block walk from the subway felt like a 5-K run. After taking three times longer than it normally would have, I arrived at the Hoffman Center late for the appointment exhausted, out of breath and hardly able to see due to the inflamed optic nerves. After a friendly greeting at the sign-in desk, they handed me several pages of paperwork to fill out. Reading the many pages of questions was yet one more struggle. Filling out page after page seemed to take forever, but that time was welcomed as my central nervous system and optic nerves were given a needed chance to recover from the walk.

After the wait, I was escorted to Dr. Hoffman's office where I shook hands with the big man and Jodi Gelfand, his Physician's Assistant. After the introductions, Dr. Hoffman asked questions about everything from my initial symptoms to my diagnosis. I gave a condensed history of my situation and told of my refusal to let MS stop me for even one second. Dr. Hoffman and Jodi Gelfand were surprised I had scheduled the appointment on a day of a Carnegie Hall concert and rehearsal. Dr. Hoffman seemed impressed with my determination not to concede, and he said I would do very well because "You have a will of iron." Upon hearing those words from this alternative medicine celebrity, there was a sudden and unexpected tingling of optimism. Three months earlier Dr. Sergott offered to write a note for permanent disability, and Dr. Markowitz did not seem to think my prospects offered much hope. For the first time since the third attack I was told I would be okay. It was clear Dr. Hoffman was basing his prognosis on my apparent determination, and this is where seeing a top-notch holistic doctor made a difference in my outlook. At the conclusion of the initial consultation, Dr. Hoffman ordered blood tests for any allergies, and his reasoning for blood tests over scratch tests is because blood tests are believed to offer far more detailed and conclusive information about possible allergies.

Several weeks later at my follow-up visit, Dr. Hoffmann and Jodi Gelfand went over my test results for allergies to forty-two food groups. They strongly advised abstaining from a long list of foods that reacted unfavorably with my blood. The list included wheat products, vegetables of the nightshade family, chocolate and all dairy. Having read *The MS Diet Book* before the third attack, I asked about Dr. Roy Swank's warning of eggs, and Dr. Hoffman disagreed, believing an egg or two per week is beneficial. Eggs are commonly thought to be in the dairy category, but they are actually an animal byproduct. Dr. Hoffman then recommended an extensive and rather expensive list of supplements. I had been somewhat hesitant about going to see Dr. Hoffman because I had been forewarned of his fees and the cost of his supplements.

Seeking his advice turned out to be a prudent decision in my battle and it was definitely money well spent.

Stacking the Deck in My Favor

At that follow-up visit with Dr. Hoffmann, he excused himself to tend to other matters, and I met privately with Jodi Gelfand who unexpectedly turned out to be an amazing source of inspiration. Her advice to "stack the deck in my favor from every possible angle" changed my entire life and future outlook. Before this one-on-one meeting, I was in a horrendous physical and mental state, and I was fighting with blind hope without any real sign for future optimism. However, it was Jodi's advice to stack the deck in my favor that was incredibly helpful; it proved to be a major turning point in the battle. Stacking the deck in my favor consisted of Jodi's five following recommendations:

1. Change my diet by eating natural food and eliminating foods that tested positive for allergic reactions.
2. Take all recommended supplements daily.
3. Exercise daily and stay in good physical condition.
4. Eliminate stress from my life.
5. Continue the Avonex® injections.

After outlining the five steps, Jodi changed my life forever when she looked me in the eye and said, "If you seriously follow these five steps, you will never hear from this illness again in your lifetime."

That stopped me dead in my tracks because I felt hope in her prophesy and those were the exact words I needed to hear. When Dr. Sergott said he had seen people in my position in perfect health one year later, it was powerful enough, but Jodi's prognosis provided not only hope, but also the needed steps that would be taken to rebuild my body and central nervous system. Time and energy would no longer be wasted being scared or thinking negative thoughts about my future. Jodi's prediction would become reality. From that moment, everything about my life would be geared to following her five steps and ensuring success. Her prophecy would have to be earned as it would not come easily, and there would be a heavy sacrificial price to pay. Thomas Edison once said, "The secret to success is 1% inspiration and 99% perspiration." A far less refined quote was often displayed on the bumper stickers of Volkswagen buses from the 1960s that read, "Gas, Grass or Ass.

No One Rides for Free." People with MS can do things to slow or even halt the progression of the disease, but what truly matters is how far they are willing to go and what sacrifices they are willing to make to achieve the result of completely beating the disease.

Before discussing each of the five recommendations, it is important to keep in mind exactly what a person is dealing with when it comes to MS. There is no blood test for the disease, so it is diagnosed from symptoms, MRIs and the process of elimination. This mysterious disease plays by its own rules, and that rulebook has not yet been made available to the public.

Jodi Gelfand's Five Recommendations:

1. Change of diet

Since the Hoffman Center had tested me for allergies to forty-two food groups, Jodi reiterated the elimination of the following foods from my diet: all wheat products, including spelt, rye, oats, barley, kamut, and particularly wheat gluten. Also on the taboo list were all dairy products, chocolate and vegetables of the nightshade family, which includes eggplant, bell peppers and white potatoes. I also eliminated all processed food and any food with chemical additives or preservatives.

Seitan is a meat substitute made from pure wheat gluten and I was almost living on it because of its texture, consistency and flavor absorbing properties that combine to make a great meat substitute. Every single food on Dr. Hoffman's forbidden list was deleted from my diet from that moment on and without a second thought. One memorable food-related event during my recovery took place after I began strictly adhering to Dr. Hoffman's dietary rules. It took place one evening when I made pasta with fresh tomato sauce for my children. Both pasta and tomato sauce were off limits, but after serving the kids, it looked and smelled so good I was salivating like Pavlov's dog. After dinner I was on solo clean up detail and I splurged with several mouthfuls of the delicious pasta, but did not swallow it. After chewing and thoroughly enjoying the taste of each bite, I leaned over the garbage and spit out every mouthful. Naturally, the level of satisfaction was equal to showering with a raincoat or engaging in the manifestation of affection while utilizing a prophylactic, but I have to admit the taste was good.

Adhering to the new food restrictions was a no-brainer because the sacrifice of foods was a miniscule price to pay for a normal life free of MS. I took the list to my own extreme, which exceeded Dr. Hoffman's restrictions, and I even began adding to his list with my own research.

2. Take all supplements daily

Taking all supplements every day became something of a ritual, and it was done every morning on an empty stomach with the reasoning my body would better absorb them without the distraction of food. I had recently discovered the Water Cure, so I chased down the supplements with my sixty-four ounces of morning water. Some of the supplement tablets and capsules were huge and it took some time to learn to swallow them, but with daily practice, I became so proficient that the horse pills were gulped down two or three at a time. The funniest part of taking all those supplements is the change of urine color. Even with the massive amount of water used to swallow them, about an hour after taking them, the color of my urine was an iridescent gold. That magical gold color was, no doubt, a reflection of the high cost of all those supplements. I mixed the daily dose of MSM powder with water but it still had an offensively bitter taste, so this is where the discipline of ignoring my complaining taste buds came into play. Along with the diet, the bitter taste was another small price I was more than willing to pay.

Dr. Hoffman's Daily List of Supplements:

- Hoffman's own daily vitamin
- 1 tablespoon of flaxseed oil
- MSM powder (an anti-inflammatory)
- CoQ10
- SAM-e
- Evening primrose oil
- Fish oil
- Grape seed extract
- Ginkgo biloba
- Calcium
- Rose hips

3. Exercise daily and stay in shape

Exercising on a daily basis was an easy one because of my yoga, my dad's teachings with his bad back, and Nolan Ryan's book, which was literally becoming my own bible. A physically fit body from a newly crafted exercise program, along with a new diet, supplements and the Water Cure would now enable the attainment of this new and highest goal to date.

4. Eliminate stress from my life

Entirely eliminating stress from my life was not a realistic goal, but I was willing to stop at nothing. Six months after the third attack I made the decision to get my own place where I could live to fight the disease without any distractions, but it would prove to have major consequences for my relationship with both of my children. For the first year on my own I lived less than one block away from my children so they could freely come and go as they pleased, but after the one year I bought a house five blocks away. Living alone did not eliminate stress but it did help in reducing it to a manageable degree. One addition that I added to my daily yoga practice during that time was Shavasana, or the Corpse Pose, which is an intensive relaxation pose that works wonders to reduce stress. This pose is a must for anyone with any stress-related issues, and that probably means everyone.

5. Continue taking the Avonex®

Taking this drug was extremely unpleasant, but I was determined to follow Jodi's advice to the letter. Being on Avonex® was challenging when traveling, and giving up one day each week was not easy. Because Jodi, Dr. Markowitz and Dr. Sergott all strongly advised it, I decided to exercise patience by giving the drug a chance to work, so I followed through with the commitment.

I left The Hoffman Center *knowing* the predictions of Dr. Hoffman and Jodi Gelfand would come true. For the first time since the initial symptoms in December of 1998, I knew I would beat MS and that it would surrender unconditionally on my terms.

January 24, 2000 was my final visit to The Hoffman Center and the last time I would see Jodi Gelfand for many years. During my recovery, I had a burning desire to tell her how well things were going and how right she had been. I knew she would be so proud and it was important for her to know just how helpful her powerful words actually were. My next meeting with Jodi Gelfand would take place fourteen years later, and it would be worth the wait.

Chapter 21

Raising the Bar - With the Bike

After two seasons of regularly biking to the train station, the rides had progressed from difficult to easy, and it was time once again for a new and higher challenge. I had always admired that one of the bass players in the orchestra commuted by bike from his home in South Jersey to the summer season rehearsals at the Mann Music Center in West Philadelphia. Here was an opportunity to raise the bar by commuting the full distance from Cherry Hill, NJ to Philadelphia on my road bike. Looking at the route on a map, it was surprisingly easy to avoid all major roads except the Admiral Wilson Boulevard, which is a main commuting route from NJ to Philadelphia, and it just happens to be equipped with a bike path along the side. Even the Ben Franklin Bridge, which crosses the Delaware River, has a separate section for bikes and pedestrians. The bike commute would increase from 3.5 miles to 11.2 miles and it would include a nearly one-mile climb to the top of the bridge.

It had been two years since my third attack and I had gained confidence to the point a practice run for this commute was not even necessary. The first time I rode the 11.2 mile commute, it took one hour, 20 minutes. After two years of doing it on a regular basis, I reduced the time to 42 minutes, my record. That may not seem like an impressive time for a distance of 11.2 miles, but this route has several traffic lights to cross the main roads in NJ, and there is a traffic light at every block in Philadelphia. Crossing the

Delaware River also involves carrying the bike up a long flight of stairs to access the pedestrian lane of the Ben Franklin Bridge.

The biggest hazard of commuting to Philadelphia by bike turned out to be the steel trolley rails in the city. One accident happened when I hit one of the rails at a wrong angle, and the other mishap was in the rain when the front tire of my bike slid out on a wet rail. Both incidents resulted in unwelcome meetings with the pavement but with only one minor injury. The first fall resulted in a hard landing on my right elbow, which was tattooed with a permanent bump as a souvenir. The second fall was on the wet rail. The bike went down so quickly that I was left with no reaction time. I was not even able to get my elbow out to break the fall. After hitting the pavement like a sack of rice, I examined my body for injuries and there was not one scratch. The reason for this stroke of good luck was my fanny pack that held a twenty-five-ounce stainless steel water bottle on each side, and one of the bottles luckily absorbed the direct impact of the fall. After seeing the bottle with a good dent from taking one for the team, it became my "lucky bottle" and it subsequently became my loyal companion on all future rides.

The challenge of biking in hot weather was solved by wetting heavy long-sleeve cotton shirts to whisk away excess body heat, but biking in cold weather would be much easier. The 11.2-mile commute was a much more strenuous workout than the 3.5 mile commute, so in temperatures above freezing the dress code required only a T-shirt and a windbreaker. Following my third MS attack, I exercised great care to avoid raising the body temperature during any workout, so training the mind to accept the wind and cold temperatures while biking allowed a strenuous cardio workout without even breaking a sweat.

One ride worth mentioning took place on a clear January morning when a temperature of 22 degrees Fahrenheit joined forces with brutally strong winds out of the west. Fighting intense wind in a car requires slightly more foot pressure on the accelerator, but fighting it on a bicycle is a different story altogether. The wind was so intense that day and I pedaled against it with all my might and managed a speed of just 8 mph on a flat road. The ride to work that morning took one hour, thirty-two minutes and I arrived at the rehearsal exhausted, but on time with only seconds to spare. There was no sweating on that memorable ride because the powerful freezing wind courteously kept my body from overheating.

Chapter 22

Preparing the Mind for Battle

Up to this point, I attributed most of my early success to discoveries I made in the areas of diet, hydration, physical conditioning and supplements. Focusing on repairing my body and tending to its needs had been immeasurably helpful, but it was now time to raise the bar intellectually as well as spiritually. The success achieved by the subjects in the MS placebo groups was high on my wish list, but there was no way of knowing how many in the clinical trials had modified their diet and lifestyle to such a radical degree. I was determined to learn their secret and it was clear that was not going to happen just from the changes I had already made. Their success obviously came from the brain and not the body, so to find the way of unlocking the power of the mind, my new area of focus would be from within.

Answers from Within

Throughout childhood, we experience certain events that will remain with us for the rest of our lives. The memories of these experiences can range from positive to traumatic, but they are part of who we are and they may be used later in similar situations. Experiences define us and they influence our future reasoning, decisions and actions. After being diagnosed with MS, I was in a complete state of denial for six months, but when denying the truth was no longer possible the decision was made to take a stand and fight the disease. In addition to the helpful things that I discovered from my own research, I began revisiting many past experiences that would help with my struggle over the next several years. MS is a unique disease because there are so many unknown variables. No one knows the cause or the cure of this particular illness; it is possible they will never be known. A great deal of mystery surrounds what may help and what may hinder, and this is where I learned from trial and error. It would be great if every one of my trials wound up with a solution, but there were unfortunate errors and some of them proved costly.

When optic neuritis first struck in February 1999, there was a one-week wait to begin intravenous steroids and that delay resulted in slight permanent vision loss in my left eye. Years later I discussed that theory with Dr. Markowitz and he disagreed, saying there is no way to be certain of that. He may be correct, but when optic neuritis struck for the second time in July 1999, I began IV steroids the next day and the vision in that eye eventually returned completely. Therefore, I remain convinced that the immediate steroid treatment was instrumental in the full and complete recovery of my right optic nerve.

It took nearly two years for the vision of the right eye to return to normal, but the left eye returned only to the point it was after my second attack. Dr. Markowitz is an excellent neurologist and has years of experience, but it is hard to argue with the results of what took place when there was no delay in starting the steroids. I have no doubt his decision to prescribe ten days of intravenous steroids was the only move, and without it there would have been serious and permanent vision loss in both eyes. At one point Dr. Markowitz marveled at how well I responded to steroids. Therefore starting them at the first sign of optic neuritis in February 1999 would have been a prudent move.

After my third MS attack I was down with one shoulder on the mat and I was about to be pinned, so the only option was to quickly come up with some way of getting out of the pin and doing a reverse. One answer was to resort to my own experiences, both good and bad, and find the wisdom gained with each one. When fighting MS it will not be enough to exercise, to make dietary changes, take western medicine, holistic medicine and reduce stress. The battle with MS will not be won fighting solely on a physical battleground because the main battle will be fought on an intellectual, psychological and spiritual front. The placebo effect is not merely happenstance, so that part of the war cannot be left to chance.

Every moment in life that has been a lesson must be put to use for the task of beating the unfavorable odds. The mind must be sharp, the body must be fit, and one must learn the ability to resort to events and lessons from the past that have been stored away in the subconscious mind. Certain events that we remember from childhood are remembered for a reason. Those events may very well be a great help during a health crisis. Our lives are filled with moments in which split second decisions are made; the soundness and the results of those decisions may not be known for some time. Thankfully, my life is made up of more good decisions than bad ones, but as a typically insecure human being I spend far more time reflecting on my bad decisions.

Chapter 23

Acting Lessons

As a typical child growing up in the 1960s, I spent too much time in front of a television set, or the "boob tube" as Dad called it. The name was appropriate because it was a black and white console television with vacuum tubes, and it required a stern whack on the side to correct its chronic fuzzy picture issue. Most of my time in front of that set was wasted, but I loved good shows and movies with great actors who had the ability to not only act a role, but to become the role. That skill would be a necessary one in my battle because the fight for my life required a total makeover of my mindset as well as my lifestyle. The actors I truly admire are the ones not limited to any one style of acting, but they are the ones who become completely different people in each role they portray.

Great actors will spend endless time researching a role. Months are devoted to learning the environment, lifestyle and mannerisms of their characters. When gearing up for the fight against MS, my desires no longer mattered. I directed everything in my life to my new acting role as the MS warrior. Diet, exercise, mental discipline and my schedule were all put to work as servants to assist in the acting of my next role.

It may seem bizarre to include a television series and movies as a source of guidance when fighting MS, but they can actually be helpful considering the inherent mysteriousness of the disease. This is not a reference to the mindless sitcoms on primetime television, but rather the shows that leave a person thinking long afterward. Some of my favorite television shows and movies are the philosophical ones that challenge the mind and get people to contemplate what is possible by thinking outside of accepted rules.

Kung Fu

During my early teen years, one of my favorite television shows was the series *Kung Fu*, starring David Carradine. My interest in martial arts attracted me to the show, but the display of martial arts in the show was weak. David Carradine did not have any background or training in martial arts to carry this aspect of the show. What sustained my interest in the show was Carradine's character, the Chinese immigrant Kwai Chang Caine. After being wrongly accused of murder, Caine fled China and drifted from town to town in the wild American west during the 1800s. His survival depended on the martial arts training and philosophical education he acquired as a Shaolin Monk in China. While growing up in China, Kwai Chang Caine studied as a Shaolin Monk, and there he developed exceptional skills in martial arts and Eastern philosophy. When difficult or dangerous situations arose in the American west, he resorted back to relevant experiences and lessons with his masters in the Temple. Of course, the script consistently had pertinent and convenient experiences of lessons from his past that provided answers and solutions to his problems of the present.

Scenes of his meditative moments from the past were actually quite helpful when thinking of ways to beat MS. One scene in particular that planted a seed in my mind took place during a lesson in the Temple. The master teaches the young Caine that development of the mind can only be achieved when the body has been disciplined. That short scene always remained with me and it was actually utilized in my battle. I knew my body had to be extremely well conditioned and prepared for the struggle I was facing. It was this mindset along with diet, yoga, weight training and biking that served as the tools to discipline my body. A disciplined and finely tuned body and successful programming of the brain, worked together to enable me to reach my goal of a total recovery.

Another of my favorite scenes from the *Kung Fu* series takes place during young Kwai Chang Caine's early interactions with his elderly blind Shaolin master. As a boy, he is unable to comprehend the master's extraordinary abilities and insight without the use of his vision. The master tells Kwai Chang Caine to close his eyes and tell of what he hears. With his eyes closed, the boy hears the nearby running water and the birds, but nothing else. The blind master then asks if he hears the grasshopper at his feet. The boy opens his eyes and watches in astonishment as a grasshopper jumps away. He asks the master, "Old man, how is it you hear these things?" and the master responds, "Young man, how is it you do not?" I found this scene to be directly applicable when it came to learning to listen to my body. Learning the signals from my body was the key to understanding the unique language of communication between the nerves and the brain. Our modern society is abundant with medications that act to mask the body's means of communicating with the brain, and the use of these medications is often self-defeating. If certain foods make a person feel heartburn or illness, it may very well be best to consider what has been ingested instead of taking medication to counter the body's message to the brain.

Movies That Inspired Me

The Matrix

"*The answer is out there and it will find you, if you want it to.*"

This quote is what Trinity the heroine tells Neo when he is searching for the answers to what is wrong in his life. This is exactly the way I felt about MS, because I was getting little help from the accepted methods of treatment, and I knew my answers were out there – just waiting for me to find them.

The Matrix was one of my favorite movies early in the recovery and I watched it numerous times. The movie is based on a science fiction comic book, but fantasy and science fiction should be taken seriously because they are creations of the imagination. The imagination is a powerful tool when fighting a disease as mysterious and unknown as MS. *The Matrix* is about a virtual world that unknowingly exists only in the minds of an imprisoned population, and the few that are fortunate to be free of this virtual prison learn and practice the necessary survival skills as they fight the restrictions of their confined world. For me the strongest message from this movie is that anything is possible if one truly believes it is possible.

Limitless

I saw this movie long after I had recovered, but the theme of this film was equally powerful and applicable. This is about a drug that enables a person to access the complete power of the human brain. After taking the drug the main character is able to recall with detail every moment from his past and is able to organize that information with the utmost efficiency. This movie touched me because we are all capable of greatly improving the power of our minds, but we do not need drugs to do so. Just as the human body is improved by changes in diet, lifestyle and exercise, combining those same changes with meditation and positive thought can sharpen the mind. Of course, these movies are fantasy and are made with blockbuster goals in mind, but the idea of a pill to unlock the power of the mind is not that farfetched.

I definitely do not have exceptional abilities of the brain, but to a large degree, I have learned to unlock the power of my mind to produce physical changes in the body. When Dr. Markowitz looked at my 2013 MRIs and said I had done the impossible, I realized that having been hit so hard and fast by MS was actually an advantage when fighting the disease. The eight months I was given to come to terms with or accept the disease was rather short, and I was forced to react with a desperate determination.

Movies That Terrified Me

MS has a unique way of instilling a debilitating sense of fear into people. The anxiety and stress before and after a diagnosis can be intense. This terrifying disease is an invisible monster that leaves behind a visible path of destruction. The victims tend to feel helpless and they are too often left trying to clean up the damage. When my third attack hit, I was consumed by constant worries and bad dreams that were painfully reminiscent of the psychological childhood trauma I experienced after seeing horror movies. My fear of the disease took me back in time to that stage of my life once again.

Three Tales of Terror

My earliest memory of a horror movie that caused emotional trauma is an old Boris Karloff movie, *Three Tales of Terror*. After watching this collection of three short stories on our old black and white console television, a constant fear remained within that made it difficult to go downstairs into our basement alone or enter any room in the house while it was dark. One disturbing incident was etched into my psyche after seeing this movie as a young child, and it happened in our house one night after dinner. My father told me to go down to the basement to get something. I told him I was too scared to go downstairs alone. Understandably, he said I was being ridiculous and yelled at me to go retrieve what he wanted. Terrified, I went down the stairs to the basement and slowly opened the door. My older brother Billy was mischievously lying in wait for me in the dark basement. He suddenly sprang out with both arms extended and screamed at the top of his lungs. I was in such a total state of fright that I wet my pants and began to cry. This memory now seems comical and there is no doubt my brother only meant fun and games, but at the time, it was extremely traumatic and there was little humor to be found.

Hush, Hush, Sweet Charlotte

This scary movie gave me several years of psychological trouble. To a child the images of a young Bruce Dern being hacked to death with an axe were so graphic that I should have refrained from seeing this film until years later when I would have been able to handle it. For quite a long time after seeing the movie, I was terrified of some mysterious person hiding behind a closed door who was ready to surprise me with a swing of an axe. At times it was literally paralyzing.

Night of the Living Dead

One of my father's favorite pastimes was a father and son movie night to see a film that one of us really wanted to watch. When I was in sixth grade he took me to see the classic horror film *Night of the Living Dead*. At that age I probably should have been over being affected by horror movies. This was not the case because I was still getting nightmares after seeing scary movies that had hit home. This latest film affected me in a bad way, far worse than the *Three Tales of Terror* and *Hush, Hush Sweet Charlotte* had several years earlier. *Night of the Living Dead* was filmed in black and white, and it lacked the special effects wizardry of today's horror films. That resulting void can leave far more to the imagination and have an even greater effect on young and impressionable minds.

The late night drive home from the theater compounded the psychological impact of the movie because my dad took the opportunity to test out his new 1971 Dodge Charger that was equipped with a 383 engine that was fed by a four-barrel carburetor. This vehicle was a performance machine and I remember him opening the throttle and reaching a speed where the dotted white line in the center of the highway looked like a solid white line. From the front passenger seat, I looked over at the speedometer that was registering a speed of 120 mph. The combination of the horror movie and that high-speed drive succeeded in putting a knot in my stomach that remained for some time.

The aftereffects of that evening were the disturbing nightmares that stayed with me for several months. When I see these films now, it is bewildering how they could have had any lasting effect. They are not the least bit scary because the acting is labored and the special effects seem amateurish. In hindsight I was far too young and impressionable for such horror movies, and it would have been better to have not seen these films until I was older.

The Shining

The last horror film that gave me nightmares was *The Shining*, which I saw just after graduating from Juilliard. This is a psychological thriller that once again touched my core, and while I was no longer afraid to go into a dark room by myself, this film left me with residual nightmares for a while. To this day I still find it difficult to watch horror films because the childhood trauma experienced from those movies still exists.

Chapter 24

Dad and His Rages

It is not my intention to portray my father as an abusive parent in any way. However, he was physically abused as a child and it is human nature to raise our children just as we were raised. He may have had a bad side but he also had a wonderful side that far eclipsed any negativity, and I have many good memories of the two of us spending quality time together.

When I was young my father would go into periodic rages, and when he did my brother and I were subjected to his ritual beatings. To receive one of these beatings we had to do something foolish and senseless as only young children can do; nevertheless, Dad always seemed ready to administer the punishment. Another time I remember wetting myself was when my father was irate over something I did. He slapped me so hard it knocked me off my feet and I lost control of my bladder.

My brother Billy is the oldest of the siblings and he bore the brunt of my father's wrath, but Billy was always tough and he firmly stood his ground with my father. I was absolutely terrified of the beatings and was never able to comprehend how my brother was never afraid. To this day I can still hear the sounds of my brother receiving his beatings while my father was screaming at the top of his lungs. While listening to my brother being beaten from the next room I felt like a Roman gladiator who was next in line, unable to see, and subjected to hearing the preceding gladiator being brutally slain.

The psychological impact of hearing Dad beating my brother was intense and my fear was compounded by not knowing when my turn would come. During those times when my brother would receive his beatings, I never once heard him cry and I was not able to understand his strength and resolve. The only time in my life that I remember my brother crying and screaming in pain was when he was very young and had a case of osteomyelitis in his leg. He was confined to bed rest and the level of pain was too much – even for him. I was no match for my brother's bravery and strength and when I received my beatings, it was my father's face that terrified me the most. My father always had issues controlling his temper but when he administered the beatings, he would totally lose what control he did have. He became so overwhelmed with anger that his face turned red and his eyes looked satanic. The fear of getting beaten by my dad was so real that even today I can still feel my pulse quicken and my adrenaline rush when I think back on it. I never came to terms with my fear until I later faced a disease that was far scarier than my dad's anger and his beatings.

It is curious how a given situation can affect two people so differently. My father's beatings had the exact opposite result of what he intended to achieve. To my brother the beatings were physical and to me they were psychological. Billy is now a successful attorney and although I have never seen him in a courtroom, people who have seen him in action say he completely takes over the entire courtroom and instills fear in the opposing legal team. The fear of my father drove me deeper into my own world and in that secluded world I had only my imagination to keep me company. It was this solitary inner relationship that no doubt helped with the development of my skills on the cello and opened the window to my soul when making music. I wish my dad were still here because I would explain what I now understand, and what he did not understand when my brother and I were so young.

When I was in seventh grade an incident took place at my middle school when I joined two other kids in kicking a hole in a newly sheet rocked wall. To this day that mindless and juvenile act of vandalism leaves me at a total loss for any explanation. Naturally I was caught in the act and taken to the principal's office where I was berated and given a three-day suspension from school, which was to commence the very next day. Terrified of the beating I would receive for my clever actions, I came up with a brilliant plan to run away from home and live happily ever after in a chicken coop in the backyard of one of my classmates. This logic-defying plan seemed viable at the time, but it was thoughtlessly driven by the intense fear of the ensuing beating.

Before moving into my new residence, the situation was luckily resolved by my neighbor, Joe Fratamico. Joe was the principal of another school in the area and he had received early notice of my situation. Joe called me over to his home and kindly proposed to quietly resolve the matter by discretely paying for the damage to the school wall. In return I would repay him with yard work. While this seemed a plausible option, the suspension from school remained an outstanding issue; it would have been impossible to hide it from my father. At that point I broke down in front of Joe and disclosed my brilliant plan to run away the next day and take up residence in my friend's chicken coop. Seeing how terrified I was, Joe said something that changed my life and it was my first lesson in standing up to my father. Joe advised me to go straight home, explain the situation to my father in front of the entire family, and do it while firmly admitting my mistake and without being afraid.

During dinner that evening I stood up and did exactly what Joe had advised, while somehow hiding my racing heartbeat and intense fear. To my surprise there was no beating, and my punishment was only an extended grounding along with chores around the house and yard. From this experience I learned there was no beating because my father sensed no fear in me. Coincidentally, Joe Fratamico's wife Barbara would come down with a case of MS years later that was not kind to her. I recall speaking about the situation with her on one occasion, but at that time I was still busy navigating my way on that Egyptian river: Denial. My father may have been abusive, but the reason goes back to the abuse he suffered at the hands of his mean-spirited and abusive mother. There is another story about my father involving Joe Fratamico that almost wipes his slate clean.

My mother is a good friend of Barbara and Joe Fratamico, and many years ago Barbara's elderly father had fallen ill. Joe came to our house to personally give our family the sad news that Barbara's father had passed away, and he was greeted by my dad who happened to be the only one home at the time. Joe told my dad what happened and asked him to relay the news to my mother. The following weekend my mom was out on the street talking with Joe when my dad came strolling over to join the conversation. With a stern look my mother chided him, "Bill, I'm so embarrassed you didn't tell me about Barbara's father!" to which my father replied, "How is he?" He not only forgot to tell my mother about Barbara's father, he forgot that he died.

While I have finally shaken most of my childhood fears, I will always be afraid of which genetic traits I inherited from my dad. My portrayal no doubt gives the impression of an abusive father, but the intention is only to illustrate my memories of fear and the lessons that enabled me to overcome the biggest fear in my life. My father definitely had issues but he was a caring, loving dad and he sacrificed a great deal in providing for the needs and future of his four children. My siblings and I all went to college without being saddled with student loans and each one of us achieved success in our respective careers. Despite my success, I will always consider myself the black sheep of the family because I am the only one who works for someone else and does not have his own business.

Many years later I read a biography of Gandhi and it helped to understand the gift my brother possessed, which is an ability to place the will of the human spirit above emotional and physical pain. A revelation occurred in August 2009 at my father's outdoor memorial service, which took place on a pier off the west side of Manhattan. My brother gave an eloquent and moving eulogy for our father, and the part that stopped time was when he said, "My father taught me not to be afraid." It was a powerful moment because my father taught me to be afraid, but he also taught me not to be afraid. This realization proved to be one more effective weapon when battling a disease. Initially I was deathly afraid of MS but the lesson my brother taught by standing up to my father, enabled me to take a stand and face a disease without being afraid.

The anxiety and emotional pain that accompany MS are intense because one never knows when the next attack will come or what surprises it will bring. In February 1999 when I was diagnosed, fear of the unknown and ending up like Jacqueline du Pré was too much to bear. After my third attack I ran scared from anything that could remotely be considered a threat to my health and the ability to fight MS, but over the next few years it became clear I had wrested control of the situation away from MS. The moment I fully realized my fear of MS was completely gone happened in August 2013, when Dr. Markowitz looked at my lesion-free MRIs and said, "You did the impossible." The tables had turned. I was no longer afraid of MS – MS was now afraid of me.

In My Own World

We all have the ability to immerse ourselves in our own world, and this skill enables us to concentrate and focus our minds to accomplish things. During my battle with MS I began to fully understand and appreciate my meditative abilities as a gift. When I was a child my father constantly got angry and yelled: "You have your head up your ass!" He used that phrase on a regular basis because I was usually in my own world and it infuriated him beyond belief. That ability to withdraw into my own world enabled me to excel at the cello, and later on it would be used once again to effectively fight and defeat an incurable illness. My wife Teresa believes I have Asperger's Syndrome or mild autism. If that is the case I am grateful and would not trade it for anything in the world.

It has been five years since my dad's passing, and that excited child inside wants to run and show him my MRIs and proudly share how I beat MS. I would explain that having my "head up my ass" was really a gift, and how it made so many things in my life possible. If that moment were to take place there is no doubt Dad would laugh and apologize the only way he knew how: by asking if I needed any money.

Dad's Back

Certain events witnessed by a child will remain vivid memories for life. One such event took place one evening when my father was carried home from work by four men and laid on our living room floor. Back then my father was slightly overweight and he struggled with chronic lower back pain, but this time he was completely debilitated by what would later be diagnosed as a herniated spinal disc. He proceeded to spend six miserable weeks in traction on our newest piece of furniture, a hospital bed in the middle of our living room. After getting out of traction, he sought the advice of no less than four orthopedic surgeons for a solution to his back trouble. Three of the doctors said surgery was the only option, but the fourth doctor said my father had two choices: he could undergo surgery or he could exercise every day for the rest of his life. My dad wisely opted for the latter and that choice offered me the opportunity to grow up seeing him perform his daily morning exercises.

This lesson in discipline would prove helpful with a teenage martial arts back injury of my own. It would be invaluable when I was faced with a deadly serious health crisis. My father's example was not just a lesson in discipline, it was a lesson that demonstrated the power of the human spirit. After years of back trouble that began at a relatively early age, my father's daily exercise regimen staved off any further back issues for the remainder of his life.

Dad's fortunes changed for the worst at the age of seventy-five when he underwent a twilight-life crisis and moved to Tucson, Arizona. This move to a place 2,000 miles away from everyone he knew was against his family's wishes, and he did it on a moment's notice. In his new environment Dad bought a single family house and told his neighbors he was several years younger than his actual age. While installing a ceiling light fixture in his new house, he fell off a ladder and landed on the ceramic tile floor. The fall, which knocked him unconscious, resulted in a compound fracture of his left leg and a severely damaged left knee. Alone when it happened, he was lucky his quick-thinking dog began barking uncontrollably at two contractors who were working outside the house next door. Sensing something wrong, they entered the house and found him on the floor out cold with the broken tibia protruding from his leg. He was rushed to the local hospital for emergency surgery where his leg was set and hardware was installed around his badly damaged knee.

My younger sister Leah, a successful personal trainer in Richmond, Virginia, promptly traveled to Arizona to collect Dad and bring him back to his family on the east coast. After several weeks, it was painfully obvious that the damage to his left knee was so extensive that a replacement was needed, so Dad reluctantly underwent the procedure. Sadly, the day of his fall from the ladder was the last time he exercised and he never even underwent physical therapy following his knee replacement. Self-pity had set in with a vengeance and Dad accepted his mortality, which greeted him a short time later. In his last few months when I would ask how he was doing, his response was always, "Just waiting to die." It was difficult to see Dad lose his spirit, passion and discipline that enabled such a good quality of life. I tried in vain to motivate him and reteach the values he taught me as a child, but it was not meant to be.

My mother would be truly disappointed and this book would be incomplete without one event related to Dad's back. Since my earliest memories I was always intensely focused on one particular 'kick' where an obsession with something would be my purpose in life for an extended period of time. This form of obsessive compulsive disorder was always present in my life and it included everything from constantly playing with G.I. Joe dolls to wearing a Superman suit under my clothes. During the time my father was incapacitated with back trouble, nothing in life existed except my cherished set of Lionel trains, and this obsession was so extreme I would sit on the floor playing with the set for hours on end, completely withdrawn from the world.

One time I carelessly left the electric transformer to the train set powered on and unattended for several hours, and it burned out. I was in a state of mourning over my loss and my loving mother could not stand to watch her obsessed child play with an inoperable train set. She promptly ordered a replacement transformer from Sears' mail order, which initiated a six-week wait for delivery. Those six weeks were agonizingly slow and the seconds passed like hours. Every day after school my greeting to Mom was, "Did the transformer come yet?" After many long weeks that magical box finally arrived, and it happened to be on the same day my dad was carried home by his colleagues.

Early in the evening he was brought into the house and carried up the stairs. As the four men were attempting to coordinate eight hands to lower him down, I ran over in an oblivious state of excitement with my long awaited treasure shouting: "Daddy, Daddy, my new transformer came from Sears!" Every adult in the room broke up with a laugh I had never heard before, and the four men carrying my father nearly dropped him. Dad later said he did not know what hurt more at that moment, his back pain or his laughter. Initially I had no idea what was funny, but eventually I saw the light. This is one of my mother's favorite childhood stories and it definitely lends credence to my wife Teresa's diagnosis of her husband's Asperger's Syndrome or mild autism.

Chapter 25

Two Early Battles That Prepared Me for War

Asthma

The late 1950s was a time when doctors actually recommended which brands of cigarettes to smoke. My mother had been indoctrinated into this club and she smoked for the full nine months while preparing my entry into the world. There is no way of proving this caused my childhood respiratory issues, but I had an abundance of breathing trouble growing up. At the age of two, a wicked case of pneumonia almost ended things, and I spent a week confined in an oxygen tent in a hospital room before finally gaining the upper hand. I have no recollection of that experience, but Mom assured me it really happened. After that, I was left with asthma that was easily triggered by certain allergies. The resulting attacks were often followed by a trip to the emergency room for a cocktail of adrenaline and epinephrine. Those attacks felt like a losing wrestling match against a large opponent who pinned my shoulders to the mat by sitting on my chest with all his weight. Every breath was an ordeal. It felt impossible to get air through my swollen bronchial tubes.

I was in seventh grade when I began studying martial arts with my next-door neighbor, and for the first time I started getting my body in shape. My brother Billy was on the high school track team, so he inspired me to start running and I noticed the cardiovascular workout was making my lungs feel stronger. The martial arts and the running were helping with my asthma, but several months later, I stumbled onto a book that would change my life forever: *The Complete Illustrated Book of Yoga*, by Swami Vishnudevananda. One thing that impressed me about this book was the beautiful dust jacket and hardcover. It is one of the most authoritative books on the subject and acquiring my own hardcover copy of the book, which had long been out of print, remained a fantasy for many years until the miracle discovery of eBay. I recently purchased another copy that was listed in "good" condition. I was disappointed when the book arrived in "fair" condition, but when I opened it, it was a delight to see it was signed by the author!

My initial draw to the book was the author's amazing degree of flexibility, and this was particularly applicable because I was constantly straining my hamstrings while practicing karate kicks. With a soft cover copy of the book, I began doing some of the yoga poses with the goal of increasing flexibility, and I also began some of the basic yogic breathing exercises. Years later, one of my favorite yoga instructors said a complete series of yogic breathing exercises provides the same benefit as running five miles, and I agree with her completely. After several months of the poses and breathing exercises, the asthma amazingly began to disappear. Yoga was therefore adopted as a lifetime companion and it would later help in the fight against MS. During my worst point with asthma, I was medicated with weekly injections and a steroid inhaler. To this day, the purpose of those injections remains a mystery, but it later became obvious the medication only served to mask the symptoms of asthma. At a relatively early age, I had succeeded in curing a chronic respiratory condition, and I accomplished it on my own without drugs or medical procedures.

Tendonitis – A Lesson in Listening to the Body

The other condition I bested was a self-created inflammation of the tendons, which was a direct result of an incorrect approach to playing the cello for many hours each day. In August 1975, I went to the School of Orchestral Studies in Saratoga, NY and heard the Philadelphia Orchestra play for the first time. It was here I had lessons with the late William Stokking, the former principal cellist of the Philadelphia Orchestra. Mr. Stokking was one of those rare people with the motivational abilities to make a person believe anything is possible, and it is no exaggeration to say he instilled those values upon me that summer. After arriving back home at the end of August my mom, who never let me quit the cello during my difficult years, wondered what had happened up in Saratoga to spur such a transformation in her son.

Suddenly I was practicing extensively for the first time, but with poor form and an extremely tight approach to playing.

After several months of overuse, the tendons in the left arm and right shoulder buckled under the strain. The pain in both arms was too much to bear and I had to stop playing for several months. During this time, I saw my family doctor, an orthopedic surgeon and even a chiropractor, but nothing seemed to help. I remember asking the orthopedic surgeon if applying heat to the arm would help, and his response was adamant: "Applying heat won't do any good because to apply enough heat to have any therapeutic value, you would have to burn the skin." I went straight home, filled a pail with scalding hot water, placed my arm in and held it there. The water was so hot that it actually burned the skin, but it did make the arm feel better.

An unexpected event that finally changed things was a visit to the home of my high school friend whose father just happened to be a family doctor. After asking his father for some advice on the matter, he had a look at both arms and asked me to move my fingers and to bend and twist each arm in different directions. He then said something that provided answers to both my cello playing and my life: "I can tell you right now there is nothing wrong with your hands and arms. The problem is with the way you are playing the cello. Playing the cello is an art, not a sport, and playing a musical instrument should be easy." This was another of those "Why didn't I think of that" moments. I had been struggling with tendonitis for months and the cause of the problem, which was right there in front of me, had been completely overlooked.

I left my friend's house determined to find the way of playing the cello that would be an art, not a sport. In the process I realized this was not something that most cello teachers could realistically help with. The answer was learning to listen to my body when it throws out warning signs and to take action long before any circuit breakers are tripped. It took a few months of rebuilding from scratch, but the tendonitis turned out to be the best cello teacher I ever had. Never mind how much this helped my cello playing, this lesson of learning to listen to the body would emerge as yet another piece of the puzzle twenty-three years later when it came to battling MS.

Chapter 26

People Who Influenced and Changed My Life

Kit Cafaro – My Mother

As a dumb kid growing up, I would have quit the cello if given the chance. In retrospect, it is difficult to understand why my mom never gave up on me. The bottom line is that my mother believed I could accomplish anything. That confidence led me to believe that anything was possible if I put my mind to it. Without the early guidance and encouragement of my mother, the cello would not be part of my life today. Without the experience of mastering the cello, it is highly doubtful that I would have had the resolve and commitment to beat MS. I was an obnoxious young teenager who constantly fought with her about the cello, and it is a miracle she never threw in the towel. My father had little patience with me and even less patience with the fact that my cello lessons consumed time and resources. He would have happily let me quit, but Mom stood her ground on this one. When I was in elementary school, Mom was so devoted to continuing my private cello lessons that she even took a babysitting job in our home to pay for the lessons. Looking back, Mom was truly visionary. She possessed and demonstrated the strength and wisdom only an exceptional mother could have.

Bill Martin

Bill Martin was the music director of my high school orchestra. During those immature and foolish years, I had much to learn because I was handicapped by a serious deficit of humility. An abundance of time and energy was wasted debating my mother about how much I hated the cello and how improved things would be if she let me quit. Years later, my mother confided she had contacted Bill Martin for advice about her extreme frustration with my attitude. She had reached the end of her limits. Luckily, Bill had seen one step further. He advised perseverance. He encouraged her not to let me quit the cello and to patiently wait for the inevitable day when I would become self-motivated. It is impossible to express how much I owe to Bill for his foresight of what would one day become reality.

Steve Zvengrowski

In eighth grade, I met Steve Zvengrowski. The student body knew Steve as Dr. Z, because of his recently completed doctoral degree in music. Our first meeting, over forty years ago, remains a vivid memory to this day. I was playing the cello in a practice room of the music wing of Hauppauge High School on Long Island, NY, when Dr. Z poked his head in the door to see the person behind the sound. He asked my name and said, "Hmmm. I'll remember that." As director of the Hauppauge High School Chorus, Dr. Z was something of a legend because of his major productions at the annual Spring Pops Concerts. Under his direction, the choral performances were always the main attraction on the program because they were complete with chorus, rock group, and full brass. This was back in the 1970's when the rock group Chicago was hugely popular. Many of the pops concerts featured their music, which proved a natural fit.

Over the next few years, I learned a great deal from Steve. I sang in the chorus, took his music theory class and participated in the Spring Pops Concerts where I played lead guitar as well as the cello. Steve believed in my potential from the moment we met, and to this day that belief remains a constant influence in my life. He once said my guitar background would be invaluable for my cello playing, but that concept was difficult to comprehend at the time. Years later, his prediction turned out to be accurate. The harmonic (chords) approach of the guitar offered a view of a larger musical picture than the melodic (single voice) approach of the cello. When I play and teach the cello, it is often from a guitarist's vantage point.

I will always appreciate everything Steve taught during the four years I was fortunate to have him as a teacher. He was extremely tough and demanding with all of his students. Though he liked me, he did not give me special treatment. During the Pops Concert rehearsals, he often pulled me aside and criticized my intonation on the cello, thus enforcing his policy of no politics when it came to achieving his high standards. Steve constantly pushed students to strive for a higher level of achievement not only in performance, but in his music theory class as well. His music theory class was very advanced. When I took music theory during my one year at Juilliard Pre-College, I was over-prepared. The music theory teacher was surprised when I was calling out answers to his questions that I had learned from Steve's music theory class. At the conclusion of a class, the theory teacher called me forward because he was curious as to how I knew so much about the subject. He was impressed when I explained the background came from my public high school music theory class.

Steve and I lost touch for several years after I graduated from Juilliard, but I managed to track him down a short time later. This was in the early 1980's, when finding people without a Google search took a good deal of time and effort. When I finally succeeded in locating him, I learned he had left Hauppauge High School and was teaching at Hartwick College, in Oneonta, New York. In 1987 when he became chair of the music department at Hartwick College and I was with the Philadelphia Orchestra, Steve invited me as a guest performer to the Hartwick College Summer Music Festival. We have remained close friends to this day and I will always value our past, present and future friendship.

What I learned from Steve more than anything was his ability to get students to excel beyond their level of capability. He constantly demanded more from the students and he was never satisfied with the result. This lesson of always striving further than one's own perceived limitations taught me well. It not only helped my undertaking with the cello, but also later helped my fight against MS. The fight against such overwhelming odds required far more than what I was capable of, so I dug down to find the motivation and fighting spirit I never realized existed. Steve Zvengrowski was yet one key piece of the puzzle that enabled me to reflect on lessons from the past, and apply those lessons to the present.

Joe Tumbarello

Often, schoolchildren fear bullying by other kids. I was no exception. However, that fear was channeled to a positive and constructive effort when I developed the inkling to learn self-defense. Our new next-door neighbor, Joe

Tumbarello, was a member of the New York City Transit Police Undercover Unit. He just happened to have a black belt in karate. Eager to maintain his formidable martial arts skills, he offered to give me karate lessons two nights per week in his house. I jumped at this unique chance to study with a man who kept people in line on the subways of New York City. Joe was definitely a person you did not want to mess with.

The best part of his lessons was his complete lack of fear, which is an important and vital mindset for a student to learn. Joe worked with me on blocking punches and kicks with the forearms and shins, and in the process, he taught me how to lose fear of physical pain. Initially my shins and forearms bruised from the repeated blocking, but over time, they grew accustomed to the blows and the bruising subsided. From this, I also learned to accept and tolerate a higher threshold for pain.

Joe stressed the importance of real life conditions during our training sessions, so we trained with a real knife that had a heavy 8-inch shiny blade. One lesson with the knife involved the defense against an overhead stab by an assailant. The defense was to quickly step to the side of the incoming overhead stab, then gain control of the knife and insert the blade in a place the assailant had not planned on. During one practice session, Joe lunged quickly from above with the knife, and I was too slow to step aside. My delayed reaction resulted in a laceration to my upper leg that drew blood, but it was not serious. I learned a valuable lesson from this minor accident. Joe believed that training with a rubber knife was a waste of time. The reality of a shiny metal blade on the street is quite different from a harmless piece of rubber in the class.

I never forgot that session with the knife, but Joe taught a more valuable lesson when I was in eighth grade. It was a lesson that would stay with me for the rest of my life. A rambunctious kid in my school classroom was seated several rows behind me. When the teacher was not looking, he shot a paper clip with a rubber band and struck my upper arm below the end of my short sleeve shirt. Angry and wanting revenge, I challenged him to a fight, which he accepted. We scheduled the fight two days later, after school. That evening, at my karate lesson I told Joe of my plans to settle the score with this boy. He had a long talk with me to discourage such plans, but he did not put his foot down and insist I call off the fight. Joe explained that karate was a discipline and not a method of revenge, and if I chose to let anger rule my life he would reluctantly help get me ready for the fight. Over the next two days, I could think of little other than Joe's words and I began to see and understand his wisdom. At school on the day of the scheduled fight, I approached the paperclip shooter and told him I would prefer an apology to a fight. He jumped at the opportunity and extended his hand with a warm smile.

At one of the karate lessons, Joe showed me a large hardcover book entitled *"This Is Karate"* by Masutatsu Oyama. The book has many captivating photos that brilliantly capture the precise moments of karate masters breaking everything from boards to bricks to ice with their bare hands. As a teenager, it was bewildering to me how the people pictured in the book could break things that were far stronger that the human body. One would expect the karate masters who display super human strength to look big and strong; but instead, they appear to be skinny and agile. Their bodies are highly developed for the skills of breaking, but the true strength is in their minds. The chapter in the book on breaking stayed with me and it would later become one more set of tools used to break MS. The displays of breaking in *This Is Karate* clearly illustrate the unlimited power of the human mind. If one can train the mind to break things considered unbreakable by the human body, then one can certainly train the mind to cure diseases considered to be incurable.

Ruggiero Ricci (1919 – 2013)

Beating MS is in many ways similar to playing a string instrument. To achieve a serious level of success they both must be broken down to a science.

During a 1979 summer festival in Vancouver, B.C., I was fortunate to have met the great violin virtuoso Ruggiero Ricci. Many had reservations about his musical tastes and his skills as a poet on the instrument, but it was impossible to argue with his technical expertise on the violin. His approach to playing the instrument was fascinating because he simplified everything and he was passionate about explaining each of his methods. That summer I sat in on many of his lessons, and he was very pleased that someone had taken such a keen interest in learning the intricacies of his trademark. During those lessons, I became a sponge that absorbed everything. At times, he actually ignored his violin students to talk to me about his theories and discoveries.

At the end of that summer, I returned to New York for my third year at Juilliard. During that time, I was fortunate to have taken three lessons from Ricci in his apartment in Manhattan. Everything learned during those lessons served me well with learning to play the cello, but the invaluable knowledge gained from him was unknowingly placed in my subconscious and used later in my battle with MS. Ruggiero Ricci had a very common-sense approach to string playing and very often it was the simplest and the most obvious things that others overlooked. When he explained his violin methods, I often said to myself, "Why didn't I think of that?" Ricci was a true child prodigy, and I can say from firsthand experience that he possessed the brilliant mind of a scientist when it came to the violin. Had he devoted the same level of thought to musical artistry that he devoted to the mechanics of violin playing, I believe he would have gone down in history as one of the greatest violinists and musicians of all time. As for the science of playing an instrument, he said three things were necessary for mastering the skills on the violin or the cello:

1. Know the fingerboard as well as the left hand positions.
2. Have a good shift technique.
3. Know how to sight read.

The fingerboard of a violin or cello has no frets and there is little to guide one in the placement of the fingertips of the left hand. High-level string playing requires near perfect intonation that is achieved by pinpoint accurate placement of the fingertips. There is a natural tendency for string players to be in uncharted territory with little knowledge of exactly where to place the fingertips of the left hand. Beginning string players demonstrate the difficulty of this skill by placing tape across the fingerboard of their instruments to act as a guide. Excelling at the violin or the cello requires years of daily practice and constant maintenance of skills. Good intonation is achieved by repeated practice to ingrain the required motor memory skills. Ricci stressed the importance of being well versed in every position and to have complete knowledge of the fingerboard. He demonstrated this skill by playing two octave scales across the four strings of the violin in each position without shifting, and he repeated this exercise in every position to cover the entire fingerboard.

A good shift technique is necessary when moving the left hand from one position to a new one. This requires intricate coordination that is simply precise timing of body movement. If a string player's shifts are not smooth and seamless, the sound of the finished product will leave much to be desired. To learn and maintain a good shift technique, Ricci recommended practicing scales with one finger. This exercise entails a shift between every note. He said many students have an inadequate shift technique, so the fastest and most direct way of rectifying that weakness is by going straight to the root of the problem and focusing only on shifting.

Sight reading is another vital skill when playing an instrument, and Ricci had this one down to a science as well. Sight reading is playing music at sight without any preparation. During my lessons, he demonstrated an obvious but overlooked approach to attaining high-level sight reading skills. He took out a book of Chopin etudes for the piano, placed it on the music stand, turned on a metronome, and began playing the upper line of one of the more difficult etudes without missing a beat. He explained the discipline of forcing yourself to keep in forward motion while sight reading. He stressed the importance of keeping the eyes ahead of where you are actually playing. This is similar to speed reading, where the eyes are physically ahead of what the brain is registering.

When I was placed in a life or death situation in my battle with MS, Ricci's lessons were constantly revisited to get beating MS down to a science. Everything was reduced to its lowest common denominator and I was determined to leave nothing overlooked. In addition to his scientific approach to the violin, Ricci was highly self-motivated and his endless drive was independent of any success in his career. I am privileged to have seen his amazing level of self-motivation and his tireless work ethic firsthand. When I watched Ricci play the violin, it truly illustrated how easy something is – once you know how to do it. Ricci had an amazing passion for the violin, and he devoted his entire life to mastering every facet of the instrument.

Ruggiero Ricci passed away in 2013 at the age of ninety-four, and I regret not contacting him to let him know how helpful those lessons were in so many areas of my life. Those lessons helped me play the cello and beat MS, and they continue to stay with me. I apply them to all areas of my life on a daily basis. I never saw Ruggiero Ricci after those lessons in 1978, but I think about him most every day and truly appreciate the knowledge and wisdom he shared during those lessons.

Sarah Chang

I first heard Sarah Chang in 1990 when she was only ten years old, and she played the first movement of the Paganini D major violin concerto with the Philadelphia Orchestra. Only eight cellos were utilized for the performances and the rotation system said it was my turn to be off, so I went out into the hall to listen. Word on the street was this child was a genuine prodigy but when her father came out on the stage during the rehearsal to assume the task of tuning her half-size violin, I had serious doubts. Nothing could have prepared me for what I heard next. As she began playing my jaw dropped because it was some of the very best violin playing I ever heard live, and her level of instrumental skill and artistry was nothing short of amazing. It was difficult to believe what was taking place on the stage because my brain was not able to comprehend what my eyes were seeing. I sat transfixed on her sheer brilliance and poetic beauty, wondering if God had chosen this child as his musical voice or if it was simply a case of superior genetics. If I spent my life practicing twenty-three hours a day, seven days a week, I could never play at her level, yet this girl was just ten years old.

Sarah Chang did not help me beat MS but she did help me regain and learn new ways to play the cello. The experience of hearing her play live when she was ten years old stays with me to this very day. Most parents of children studying an instrument dream of their child being a prodigy, but a true child prodigy is a rarity. Sarah Chang was a true child prodigy in every sense, and hearing her play when she was only ten years old was one of the foremost musical experiences in my life. Seeing her play live at age ten was one thing, but watching her development over the years was an even greater privilege. Many child prodigies do not last because the intense professional pressures placed on young children are unnatural and abnormal. Children need to live a normal childhood. When a young child assumes the role of a successful concert musician, a necessary stage of that child's life is missed. Most adults would be unable to handle the intense pressure career of a solo violinist, yet this demand is too often placed upon young children. Pre-teens are generally not capable of being self-motivated, so the necessary motivation required to nurture a prodigy's development comes from the parents. When a young child shows truly rare and exceptional musical skills, the parents often assign the child their future profession and the child has no say in the matter.

As a cellist with the Philadelphia Orchestra, I have had the opportunity to watch Sarah Chang's development on a regular basis, and I often wondered how this remarkable child prodigy would cope with the stressful adult life of a concert artist. Sarah is among the truly exceptional cases where a legitimate child prodigy successfully made the transition to a mature artist. To watch and listen to Sarah play today as an adult is fascinating because in addition to her artistry on the violin, she displays wisdom with a deep understanding of show business. Classical music can be a difficult product to sell because audiences want to be intellectually stimulated, entertained, dazzled, humored and educated - all with the highest level of instrumental skills and musicianship. Sarah exhibits insight into all those requirements not only with her violin, but also with her concert attire and her physical presence and smile on the stage.

Playing a musical instrument differs from athletics because children can develop accomplished instrumental skills long before the body has developed. For a young child to play a musical instrument at concert performance level, the brain must have an exceptional ability for coordination and motor memory skills. When it comes to athletics, a finished product cannot precede the development of the body. One does not see a child prodigy throwing a baseball at 100 mph, just as one does not see child prodigy opera singers.

Sarah Chang was very helpful during my recovery because I found her to be a constant source of inspiration. My thinking was if a ten-year-old could do it, so can I. Sarah Chang could very well be on my list of people who have done the impossible, because ten-year-old children do not play the violin at such a high level. Many of the things I was able to do on the cello prior to the vicious attack of 1999 were affected because the pathways used by my brain to control the muscles were permanently changed. Thankfully, when a door closes, a window opens somewhere else. That belief left open the possibility of finding new and improved ways of playing the cello. It allowed my brain to find new and more efficient ways of using the muscles. To play the violin at Sarah Chang's level, it is not necessary to go running or lift weights because the violin takes a fraction of the physical strength that sports require. I came to the realization that my fingers, hands and arms were capable of playing at Sarah's level, but my brain was the roadblock.

People who truly excel at a skill or profession make it look easy, and it appears easy to others because they have found and understand the easier way of doing it. When Sarah Chang played so brilliantly at age ten, she simply stood in one place and did not move about the stage. Her face remained expressionless and she moved only what was needed to play the violin. The same can be said for the legendary Jascha Heifetz on the violin and Emanuel Feuermann on the cello. Many videos of Heifetz exist but there are only two of Feuermann.

During my recovery, one of the goals was to learn from Sarah Chang and unlock the secrets of how this child was able to play the violin at such an extraordinary level. Years ago, I had a Korean cello student whose mother was a busy doctor that was unable to bring her son to a lesson. A Korean woman that I did not know drove him to my house; she sat there intently listening to the entire lesson. At the conclusion of the lesson the woman said in broken English, "You are a very good teacher. Would you teach my eight-year-old son?" I explained that my busy schedule did not allow for any new students, but the truth was I had no interest in teaching an eight-year-old child.

At my student's next lesson, his mother informed me that the woman at the previous lesson who wanted cello lessons for her eight-year-old son was none other than Sarah Chang's mother. That was definitely one of those moments in life one never forgets. I have since gotten to know Sarah Chang and even had the privilege of playing chamber music with her on one occasion, but we never discussed my illness or how helpful she was during my recovery. I see her once every season when she appears as guest soloist with the Philadelphia Orchestra, so one day I may have the chance to bring her up to speed on my history. I would be most curious to hear her thoughts on exactly what enabled her to play at such a high level at such a young age. Only time will tell.

Jon Vickers - The Legendary Canadian Tenor

After auditioning for the Metropolitan Opera Orchestra cello opening in June of 1983, I was disappointed to have not been picked as the winner as most people who have taken auditions can understand. However, I was one of three finalists and getting that far in an audition with the Met certainly had its benefits. Someone from the Met called me after the audition and asked if I would be available as an extra cellist with the orchestra when the season began in September of 1983, so naturally I was delighted. Over the next few months, I played with the Met Orchestra and learned some of the great operas, but one of the best things about that experience was hearing some of the truly great singers of the time.

About seven months after I began playing with the Met Orchestra, I was walking on West 72nd Street near West End Avenue, and I happened to witness a car accident. It did not seem like a serious mishap and there were many people gathering around the scene, so I kept on walking. The next morning I received a phone call from Eddie Sodero, an older cellist at the Met who had taken me under his wing when I began working there. Eddie asked if I was available to play Richard Wagner's *Die Walküre* with the Met that evening and for the remaining performances that week. Then he asked if I would be available to join them for the upcoming seven-week tour of the United States. At that time, I had no regular job and very little money, so I obliged without revealing any excitement. It was highly unusual to be hired for so much work on such short notice so I inquired as to the reason behind it. He told me that Jerry Kagan, a cellist with the Met Orchestra, had gotten into a car accident on 72nd Street after exiting the West Side Highway. This turned out to be the accident I had witnessed the previous night. I was called to fill in for Jerry because he had broken his collarbone on the seatbelt.

As a formality, Eddie Sodero asked if I had ever played *Die Walküre* before. Being new to the Met, I was unaware of a Met rule that subs were not allowed to perform an opera unless they had rehearsed it or had performed it somewhere else. At that moment, I made a split decision and told him I had played it before. After a doubtful moment of silence he asked with a rather harsh tone, "Where?" I told him it was with an opera company in Virginia when I used to teach down there. There was another momentary pause and I could hear his wry face when he said, "All right. Well come in anyway." In the business world, there is a saying that it pays to advertise. In this case, I was lucky to have opted not to advertise.

The operas I performed with the Met over the next few months included Verdi's *Don Carlo* and *La Forza del Destino,* Wagner's *Lohengrin*, Mozart's *Don Giovanni*, Puccini's *La Boheme* and *Manon Lescout*, and Britten's *Billy Budd* and *Peter Grimes*. One of the great experiences of playing at the Met was hearing the legendary Canadian tenor Jon Vickers sing the leading roles in *Die Walküre* and *Peter Grimes*. *Die Walküre* was sung in German but when he sang the role of *Peter Grimes,* I was able to follow every word because it is in English, and a good deal of the role is sung alone without the accompaniment of the orchestra. The lesson learned from Jon Vickers as Peter Grimes was not that he sang the role of Grimes, but that he became Peter Grimes. During the opera I truly felt his pain, torment and anguish. After my time at the Met, I never gave much thought to Vickers. When I came down with MS, my vivid memories of him would be yet one more effective weapon in my arsenal against a merciless opponent.

As it turned out, I did not just act the roles of Nando Parrado, Nolan Ryan, Bobby Fischer and Lance Armstrong. I became those people and I would emerge victorious just as they did because I was each one of them in every sense. Following Nando's example, "I became a survival machine." Nolan

Ryan said, "That mound is my domain, and for me to be effective I had to be aggressive." I was Bobby Fischer when he said, "I liked to watch my opponent squirm." I was the cyclist Lance Armstrong who said, "Cancer (MS) picked the wrong person."

The Piccolo Player at the School of Orchestral Studies

During the summer of 1976, I attended the School of Orchestral Studies in Saratoga, NY, for the four-week summer program. At the end of the program, the student orchestra always performs one major orchestral work, and that year it was the Symphony No. 4 in F Minor by Tchaikovsky. The third movement of this symphony has a very fast piccolo solo that is so difficult that even the best professional piccolo players find it problematic. The student who played piccolo in the orchestra that summer was good and she taught me a lesson that stayed with me every day since.

In a practice room, which was anything but soundproof, she repeatedly drilled that solo with a metronome for several hours each day. In the process, she made the other students quite jealous. The students were getting tired of hearing her repeated practice of the solo, and some began talking about her unfavorably, with the hope she would falter at the final concert. Nevertheless, at the concert she played confidently and perfectly, and without the slightest hint of self-doubt. From her example, I learned the importance of having a goal and the perseverance to devote anything and everything to achieving that goal. It is a rarity to see someone in their teens so intensely disciplined and self-motivated, but this girl selflessly sacrificed many social activities at a point in life when social interaction and acceptance is a top priority for most.

Dr. Glenn Newell

Dr. Glenn Newell and I first crossed paths in May 2005 on the Philadelphia Orchestra's tour of Asia. Dr. Newell had recently accepted the position as the orchestra's overseas physician. On his first tour, his wife Ana and their five-year-old daughter, Isabel, accompanied him. We became acquainted when Isabel saw my impression of Donald Duck, and from that moment, she knew me as Mr. Duck. Isabel apparently took a shine to that impression, because after returning home from the tour she became my youngest cello student. It is prudent for an orchestra to bring its own doctor when traveling overseas because our past tours have seen musicians sidelined in foreign lands with various health issues that have included heart attacks, broken bones, food poisoning and even appendicitis. Although I met Dr. Newell six years after being diagnosed, his advice and medical care have been immeasurably helpful. I find him to be a fascinating individual because we share many interests, and the main one is a love for cycling.

One day on the tour, we were having a casual conversation and the subject of my MS came up. Dr. Newell was extremely interested in the story of my recovery because at that time he was creating a DVD project called *Music in Medicine,* which explores a link between the two art forms. The source of his passion is obvious because he plays a mean saxophone and loves all types of music, from classical to classic rock. When Dr. Newell asked if I would give a filmed interview for the project, I was hesitant but nervously agreed. By 2005, my health and cello playing had come back in a big way, but I was still in a state of denial about the MS. At that point, I was telling people in the orchestra I had suffered from a mysterious and unexplained illness, and MS was an obvious misdiagnosis.

The interview, which is on the DVD, was filmed on the tour and it unexpectedly turned out to be very helpful because it was a badly needed dose of emotional therapy. There is something about speaking in front of a camera that liberates a person to open up. During the interview, I felt an unexpected freedom to say things I had kept bottled up. Without any realization, I suddenly felt free to open up and come clean about the seriousness of my situation with MS. During the filming, painful emotions surfaced and I nearly broke down crying as I told of my struggle. At that moment it was clear that, because I had never been to therapy, I had kept everything buried inside for the previous six years. Therefore, this was the long awaited and needed opportunity to be open and honest about everything. It was also a time for me to come to terms with and accept what had happened.

During the three-week tour of Asia, I was fortunate to not see Dr. Newell as a patient, but we did spend a good deal of time getting to know each other and exchanging ideas. His skills as a doctor were impressive, but his openness to ideas and his ability to think outside the box were the reasons he became my primary doctor after the tour. Trust between a doctor and patient is a necessity and I knew Dr. Newell could be trusted in every sense.

Following the *Music in Medicine* interview, Dr. Newell and I had a conversation about diet and he shared his theories on the needs of the human body and the hazards of consuming too much of any one thing. One particularly helpful thing Dr. Newell mentioned is his belief of the human body's requirement for sodium. The FDA recommends limiting the daily intake of sodium at 2,500 mg, but Dr. Newell believes the human body needs only a fraction of that amount. In fact he believes the body's needs are far less than that per day. Keep in mind that sodium intake adds up quickly. For example, one slice of commercial bread contains 170 mg of sodium and that is before anything is put between two slices of that bread, such as lunchmeats, cheeses and spreads. Clearly, it is very easy to over-consume sodium. WebMD lists the five saltiest meals in restaurants and I find it shocking.

Once the human body's basic sodium requirements are met, the body is distracted by the task of ridding itself of any excess. My customized diet was formulated with the goal of not distracting the body from dealing with the primary and formidable task at hand – beating MS. This approach was applied to the mind as well as the body because a simple healthy diet consisting of small portions helps the sharpness in the mind as well as the body.

Even though Dr. Newell is my current doctor, I rarely see him as a patient. Most people would advise routine tests for health issues that are common for a fifty-seven-year-old male. The main reason behind my decision to forego routine medical tests is the *Okinawan Centenarian Study*. In many ways, I have adopted the lifestyle of the subjects in the study who were all over the age of 100 and in perfect health.

It is always fascinating when two people who are highly accomplished in their field can see things so differently. When I asked Dr. Markowitz his theories behind unexplained placebo group success, he felt the brain actually produces a chemical that makes changes in the body. When Dr. Newell was asked the same question, his theory on the matter was different. Dr. Newell does not believe a chemical that is made by the brain achieves the placebo effect, but he feels the brain somehow consciously sends signals to the muscles to act in a healing capacity. It will never be possible to determine which theory is correct, but the placebo effect certainly comes from the brain, which is basically a computer that can be programmed to perform specific tasks. This is an example of the importance behind getting information from different sources and using the information to come up with one's own system. Dr. Sergott, the Director of Neuro-Ophthalmology of Wills Eye Hospital in Philadelphia, was right when he said there was no way of knowing exactly which of the many things I did was responsible for my complete recovery. In fact, he believes it was the culmination of all the things that were done.

During the years I have known Dr. Newell and the few times I have seen him as my doctor, there has not been one occasion when I saw him about an issue related to MS. In all of his years of practicing medicine, Dr. Newell cannot recall a single case where someone has made a miraculous recovery from MS, with the exception of my case. I have little doubt Dr. Newell believes there is some connection between music and my healing. One humorous encounter with Dr. Newell took place when I saw him as a patient; I was experiencing difficulty staying awake during orchestra rehearsals. After checking me out and deciding there was nothing wrong, he asked, "What time do you go to bed at night?" Without a second thought, I replied, "Usually 1:30 am to 2:00 am," to which Dr. Newell replied, "Why don't you start going to bed earlier?" He then directed me to the receptionist to give her the office visit copay.

Chapter 27

The Story of My Cello

Bill Golz was not among those who beat an incurable illness, survived a life-threatening situation in the wilderness, pitched a baseball 100 mph or played an instrument at a superhuman level. He was an exceptional soul, an inspiration, my spiritual guide and a person who changed my life forever.

In 2006, I was invited to play a cello recital at Whitehorse Village, a retirement community in Newtown Square, Pennsylvania, with Luba Agranovsky, a truly remarkable pianist I have had the privilege of performing with since 2003. The one-hour recital included the Sonata No. 3 for cello and piano, Opus 69, by Beethoven, and the Hungarian Rhapsody, Opus 68, a cello showpiece by the great cellist and composer David Popper. The performance was well attended and afterward several residents of Whitehorse Village approached and congratulated us. Then an elderly man shuffled forward, shook my hand and smiled, "Son, you play beautifully," to which I cheerfully replied, "Thanks so much." With a serious face, he continued, "I have an old cello, would you like to see it?" It was hard to imagine that anyone living in a retirement community would just happen to have a fine old cello lying around, so I perfunctorily replied, "Sure, I would love to." Luba and I had carpooled to the recital and she was busy talking to members of the audience so she told me to go ahead and see the cello.

I followed Bill to his condominium in the complex, and he invited me into his home. He then went to the closet and pulled out an old beat-up cello case that looked rather sad. After unzipping the case, he opened it and what I saw next almost stopped my heart. It was impossible to guess the maker of the instrument, but it was clear the cello was old, most likely Italian, and in pristine condition. I stood there motionless, mesmerized by the sheer beauty of the instrument, and Bill said, "Would you like to play it?" At a loss for words and unable to speak, I simply nodded my head. Then I took the cello out of the case, pulled out the endpin, tuned it and began to play. What I experienced next was the closest I have ever been to an out-of-body experience. The cello was nothing short of phenomenal as it was effortless to play, and it was by far the best cello I had ever played in my life. I played movements from Johann Sebastian Bach's unaccompanied cello suites and excerpts from several cello concertos. All the while Bill just sat on his couch listening with a smile that never once left his face.

Suddenly I looked at my watch and realized this great cello had completely stopped time, and poor Luba had been left waiting in the main hall, so it was time to pack up. When I stood up, Bill looked at me and said the words I will never forget, "You know, when my time comes I don't want to see this cello wind up in my daughter's attic. I want to see someone like you have it and take care of it." This was yet another of those moments in life that took my breath away. As it turned out, the cello was made in 1816 in Venice, Italy by the instrument maker, Giancinto Santaguiliana.

A quick primer with old Italian string instruments: they are rare and are cherished the same as any other works of art. These instruments were traditionally expensive, but the Japanese bubble economy of the 1980's began to catapult the price of the instruments out of the reach of the people who were meant to play them. At that time, Japan had developed an insatiable love for classical music and wealthy Japanese investors began buying up old Italian string instruments. This effective combination was responsible for driving the instrument prices into an upward spiral that never ceased. To make matters worse, a disturbing trend began where these rare instruments were being removed from circulation among musicians, only to be placed in the hands of collectors where they were put on permanent display in glass cases. At the point in my career when I should have acquired an old Italian cello, it was already a pipe dream because the price was well beyond my reach.

When those thirty magical minutes with Bill Golz and the experience with that great cello concluded, we exchanged phone numbers and I returned to the auditorium to get poor Luba, who had been unhappily waiting for over an hour. However Luba has the patience of a saint, and she was excited when I told her all about the cello. Over the next few years, Bill and I became good friends, and I visited him on a regular basis. I always sent him postcards from our overseas Philadelphia Orchestra tours, and he always appreciated receiving them.

It was February 27, 2009, the day after my surgery for a depressed tibia plateau fracture that was the result of a skiing accident. I was doing my best not to wallow in misery. I was attempting to enjoy my surroundings in the Rocky Mountains of Colorado from my hospital room window. From my bed, I was trying to enjoy a good view of Vail Mountain, the geological and recreational wonder that worked its magic on my leg. Suddenly my cell phone rang and it was Bill Golz with a sense of urgency I had never before heard in his voice, and he needed to talk to me in person about "something very important." I briefly explained my predicament and said I would return home in a few days, and paying him a visit would be at the top of my list.

Two days after returning home, I embarked on the one-hour drive to Whitehorse Village in Newtown Square, PA, to visit Bill Golz. I drove there by myself, and I was clearly in no condition to be operating a vehicle. For the duration of the drive, the pain from the injury and the surgery was intense. In addition, my leg was quite swollen and keeping it elevated while driving was not a viable option. Mr. Tough Guy had decided to forego any medication for the pain because pain can be controlled with the mind. However, in this case the mind seemed to be in a losing battle with the pain, which made focusing on the road extremely difficult. After exiting Interstate 476 to go south on Route 1, the pain was so intense and distracting that I exited south onto the northbound lanes of Route 1, and proceeded to drive the wrong way on a major six-lane highway. Suddenly a wall of cars with flashing headlights and blaring horns was headed right for me, but I managed to pull over on the shoulder and breathe a sigh of relief for not killing anyone or being killed in the process

When I finally arrived at Bill's place unscathed, he had been moved to a private hospital room to deal with his own health issues. Bill began by telling me he was not well and was no longer able to play the cello. Because of his declining physical condition, he explained the time had come to part with the cello, which had been his loving companion for most of his life. There was a sadness in his voice when he announced it was time for me to have the cello. He had decided to sell the cello to me for a price that was actually closer to giving it to me than it was to selling it. In addition to the cello, he included his two English cello bows, one made by John Dodd and the other by W.E. Hill & Sons. I had no idea exactly what the cello was worth, but I knew it had to be far more than what he wanted. I immediately offered to give him what I had in savings as a down payment and said I would get a loan for the remainder, but Bill said not to worry about the loan because he had already decided to finance a loan over three years at zero percent interest. He asked about my ability to pay it off in three years, and I told him it would not be a problem. At that point, Bill produced several contracts to transfer ownership of the cello.

After signing all the papers, Bill's emotional side overtook his business side and he told of his countless sleepless nights spent wondering what would become of the cello after he was gone. It was obvious Bill had put a great deal of time and thought into securing a home for this great cello in the hands of its next caretaker. Bill was an engineer by trade and not a professional cellist, but he was admirably skilled on the instrument and his love for both music and the cello was unrivaled. He taught me all too well that we do not own things in life, but we are privileged to use things only during our time on this earth. All possessions are passed on to others at some point, and Bill knew this was the moment for this great cello. A cello, especially a fine, old one is not a material possession, but a work of art and a living being with a soul that needs constant love and care. This magnificent instrument has not only become my companion, but it has become a spiritual presence in my life.

After Bill appointed me caretaker for the cello, I visited him on a regular basis and played his favorite cello works. Each time, he listened with that happy smile that I remembered from the very first time I played his cello. Following each private recital, we went out to his favorite restaurant for lunch. The highlight of playing for him was in March 2010, when I played the Dvořák Cello Concerto with the Lower Merion Symphony in Merion, PA. Before the concert, I picked up Bill at his residence, brought him to the concert, had dinner with him afterward and then drove him back home. During the performance, he sat near the front. From the stage, I could see his face glow with joy as he listened to his cello in the leading role of one of the greatest cello works ever written. While playing the concerto, I felt that familiar joy from seeing him smile while listening, which once again elevated me to the out-of-body experience I felt the very first time I played his cello.

Each time I visited Bill, it became progressively more difficult to see his state of health in a gradual decline. Death is part of life but part of me hoped the rules could be bent or broken in Bill's case. I played for Bill while he was confined to his bed with a broken arm due to a recent fall. Bill was uncomfortable and in pain, but when I began playing the first Bach Suite in G Major, that warm smile from our first meeting illuminated his face and his spiritual presence transcended his failing physical body. He offered an opinion that I was trying too hard while playing, and his assessment was no doubt accurate because I was subconsciously trying to change what was in store for him. An eerie feeling persisted that this might be the last time we would see each other, and that it might be the last time he would hear this magnificent cello. Before leaving, I leaned over his bed, gave his frail body a hug and thanked him for teaching me so much in this life. He smiled, and said: "I'm so glad I found you."

Several weeks passed since we had been in touch, and on Oct 7, 2013, I dialed his number and was surprised when a woman answered. After asking to speak with Bill Golz, the woman sounded preoccupied and said it was not a good time, but when I said my name, her voice brightened and sounded happy. It was Bill's daughter Nancy, who had been by his side for the last few days because his time was approaching. I asked if it would be all right to come play for him one last time, but Nancy was not sure he would last. Nevertheless, we set up a time during my first free period, which was two days later. On Thursday, October 10, I texted Nancy first thing in the morning and she replied saying Bill was in and out, but knew I was still coming. I had two commitments that morning, a rehearsal for a memorial service to bid farewell to Virginia Halfmann, a former violinist of the Philadelphia Orchestra, and a dress rehearsal for the orchestra's subscription concert that night. I texted Nancy with my 1:15 pm ETA, and headed over following the orchestra rehearsal. It was such a good feeling I would get to see Bill and play this cello for him one last time, but when I was five minutes away Nancy texted, "My father just passed away. We were so close." It was such a sad moment and so many difficult emotions ran through me. I tried to stay focused on driving, but the tears in my eyes made it difficult. I texted back saying I would still like to come and Nancy said it would be great.

When I arrived, Nancy and several of Bill's close friends greeted me with the hope I would play something on the cello in his memory. When I began to play Bill's favorite Suite No. 1 by J.S. Bach, Nancy listened with tears in her eyes. Although Bill had left the physical world, I felt the presence of his spirit in the room. With my eyes closed, I could see that magical smile on his face as he listened along with everyone who was present. I know he will always be there smiling when I play this great cello.

There was no mention of it in our legal contract, but Bill asked that I never sell the instrument to the highest bidder. He wanted to know that when my time came, I would find the next caretaker for this cello just as he had done.

Bill, do not worry, I will fulfill your wish, just as you taught me. I will always miss you, and I know you will be with me as my guide when it is my time to find the next person worthy of being the caretaker for this great cello. You have forever changed my life in ways you never could have imagined. I am so glad we found each other.

Chapter 28

The Elusive Higher Goal

"Always aim for the moon, even if you miss, you'll land among the stars."

- W. Clement Stone

The people who were my guides may be credited with accomplishing impossible feats and they all had one thing in common: each one strived for a constant higher goal and not one was satisfied with their accomplishments. Every individual remained "hungry" and was never content to sit back and live off the interest of success. To succeed in accomplishing the impossible one must constantly replace achieved goals with new and higher goals. Soon after returning home from the hospital in 1999, I immediately set several goals, and as each objective was successfully met the bar was immediately raised for an even greater challenge. During that ten-day stretch on intravenous steroids I was rendered physically useless and was confined to the bed. At that point reading was a forlorn hope and I lacked the emotional capability to listen to music or the radio. While lying in bed day after day I dreamed of riding the bike once again and the goal was set to do so as soon as it would be physically possible. Getting that first ride in was top priority, so I did not wait for it to happen. Instead I made it happen at the earliest possible moment after getting home from the hospital.

Going on my first overseas tour after getting out of the hospital was a major challenge to say the least, but I was not going to back down. Many difficult issues would have to be addressed in advance, and first on the list was my new MS-fighting diet. Overseas tours pose a challenge for anyone on a restricted diet for several reasons, and the first one is foreign language. Language barriers often present a challenge, so ordering at a restaurant can often mean a step into the twilight zone. On several overseas tours in the past I have placed specific orders in restaurants and received the chef's surprise.

After much research and customizing a dietary plan, my solution was simple: Eat only organic food whenever possible, and do not eat food that was not meant to be digested by the human body. I assembled a diet as a result of blood and allergy tests performed by Ronald Hoffman, M.D., and based it on the following:

- *The Multiple Sclerosis Diet Book*, by Roy Laver Swank, M.D., Ph.D. and Barbara Brewer Dugan
- *The Okinawa Program,* by Bradley J. Willcox, M.D., D. Craig Willcox, Ph.D. and Makoto Suzuki, M.D.
- *The Okinawa Centenarian Study*
- *Nolan Ryan's Pitcher's Bible*, by Nolan Ryan and Tom House
- *The Complete Illustrated Book of Yoga*, by Swami Vishnudevananda

My diet was devised from the above books and my own trial and error, and it seemed to leave few opportunities to eat in restaurants in foreign countries for three weeks. Therefore I made the decision to restrict myself to the new diet and eliminate eating in restaurants while on tour. How does one eat for three weeks on a tour of Europe without eating a single meal in a restaurant? If there is a will there is a way. Resorting to my previous backpacking experience, I compiled a list of things to bring on tour to prepare my own meals.

- One electric hotplate
- One 220v to 120v power converter
- One lightweight set of stainless steel backpacking pots
- Organic grains, beans and peas brought from home
- A good quality portable water filter

My new diet on the 2000 Philadelphia Orchestra tour of Europe was not easy, but it was a success because all my meals were prepared right in my hotel room. An electric hotplate is a marvel of simplicity because it is nothing more than a heating coil burner mounted on a metal box. Electrical current in Europe is 220 volts, so a power converter was used to power the 110 volt burner. It felt somewhat strange to be preparing backpacking trip meals in five-star European hotels, but the hotplate and power converter worked flawlessly for the three weeks. The grains were made first and it was always either quinoa or brown rice. First the grains were rinsed thoroughly then placed in a pot with double the amount of cold filtered water. Once the grains were brought to a boil I removed them to start cooking something else on the single burner. Surprisingly, some of the dishes were actually quite good. One of my favorites was split pea soup made with peas that had been soaked in water for eight hours before cooking.

In Europe I shopped at local grocery stores for onions, carrots, celery and other vegetables that were a welcome addition in the soup. I remember being unable to get organic produce, so this was one area where going conventional was the forced option. Luckily the hotel rooms all had mini-bar refrigerators, so I emptied them out to make room for the produce and food I had prepared. Since Avonex® had to be refrigerated, I made a request for every room with a refrigerator in advance. On the long overseas flights the three doses of Avonex® had to be refrigerated, so the flight attendants were kind enough to supply dry ice for the insulated pouch I carried.

Raising the Bar - The Principal Cello Auditions

In August 1999, I sat motionless in the examination chair of Dr. Sergott's office at Wills Eye Hospital when he made the announcement about my life on permanent disability. Even though I was a complete physical mess, there was no way I was going on disability. Since it was not an option, it was clear that some highly motivational goal was needed to get me moving forward. The immediate and most important goal was to return to work in six weeks for the start of the Philadelphia Orchestra 1999 – 2000 season. Rejoining the orchestra that September was an incredibly difficult undertaking, but having done so meant a major initial goal was achieved. I succeeded in going back to work and was proud to have taken only one week of sick leave during my entire first season back. Missing that one week was not a matter of choice, but a necessity caused by a mysteriously infected right elbow that temporarily put the brakes on my triumphant return. There had been no injury to the elbow, the culprit turned out to be immunosuppressant complications from the massive doses of intravenous and oral steroids.

As difficult as that season with the orchestra was I managed to keep going, and over the next few months everything that was stripped away slowly began showing signs of returning. My eyesight, the use of my hands, my strength, stamina and cello playing were all improving slowly with each passing day. In less than seven weeks after getting out of the hospital, I reached my goal of returning to the orchestra. Now it was time to aim higher for a bigger challenge, and the bar would be set higher for a more demanding and difficult goal.

"Do better if possible, and that is always possible."

- Jean-Marc Vacheron

The Auditions

After getting out of the hospital in 1999, I was home lying in bed getting pumped full of methylprednisolone and fantasizing about getting back on the bike. Being on a bicycle is the first true sense of freedom a child will ever experience, and being trapped in an MS/steroid prison made me long for the taste of that freedom once again. Even more than simply wanting to get MS under control, I began feeling the desire to beat the disease entirely. This is where my admiration for Lance Armstrong came in, because I wanted to do what he did. I was determined to make a complete recovery from a disease that should have beaten me, and go on to win a major competitive event. It was obvious that winning a competitive athletic event was not an option, but there was a more realistic option, which was to win a race of a different nature: a principal cello audition!

As a member of the Philadelphia Orchestra, I belong to the American Federation of Musicians (AFM), which is the musicians' union. They publish a monthly list of openings in the orchestras, and while browsing the job openings I saw my next goal - the Principal Cello vacancy in the Los Angeles Philharmonic. This new goal would serve two purposes: I would start seriously practicing, and I would win the audition and be Lance Armstrong of the cello. Preparing for a major orchestra audition is a huge undertaking; anyone who has taken one will tell you exactly that. To take an audition in my poor state of health presented formidable challenges. The use of my hands was extremely limited, and I had been a stranger to the audition scene for fifteen years. It is much easier for young conservatory graduates to win auditions because they have the luxury of being able to devote all of their time to the task with no distractions. My situation was different because I had a full-time orchestra job, owned a house, had two children, was teaching cello lessons and was involved in many other time-consuming activities. Despite all of those challenges I made up my mind to become the Lance Armstrong of the cello where I would come back from the abyss and win a principal cello audition.

The Los Angeles Philharmonic Principal Cello Audition

When there is an audition on the calendar, there is no shortage of motivation. I mailed my resume to the L.A. Philharmonic and because I was a member of the Philadelphia Orchestra, they extended an invitation to the audition. The die was now cast so I began practicing very slowly and seriously, focusing on the most basic cello skills. The trick was to rediscover the mindset of what I had done at the age of sixteen when I became self-motivated with the cello, but things were more difficult at this point due to the limited use of my hands. This new challenge forced me to reexamine my entire approach to the instrument, and to constantly look for new and improved ways to play. Every movement of the arms, hands and fingers went under the magnifying glass in search of optimum efficiency. The slate had to be wiped clean because I was literally relearning to play the cello from the beginning, so everything I had previously learned had to be cast aside. I reacquired the mindset I had when I first got serious about the cello to increase the efficiency of my practice time. Attention was focused on how little effort was required for every note on the instrument, and once again several hours each day were devoted to scales of all forms. Because it had worked so well previously, the time on scales consisted of the basic scales, broken thirds, the arpeggios and the scales in double stops (playing two notes at the same time).

In addition, a good deal of time was spent each day studying the videos of Jascha Heifetz because of his unmatched level of effortlessness when it came to playing a string instrument. I had listened to his recordings for several years before ever seeing a video of his playing, and the first time I saw footage of his playing, it did not make sense. On his audio recordings his violin screams with passion and excitement, but on video he looks uninvolved because he does not move one muscle more than is necessary to play the violin. When Heifetz played he never made faces and there was no dancing about the stage. He stood motionless and all his unseen efforts were focused on only the mechanics of playing the violin. My focus was to understand and apply the same approach to the cello, which is ergonomically a more natural instrument to play than the violin. The violin is held up high by the left hand that is unnaturally twisted, and the cello is played with both arms down and in a far more natural position.

I also devoted a good deal of time once again to the etudes by the cellist and composer David Popper (1843 – 1913). His famous book, *The High School of Cello Playing*, is a collection of 40 etudes, and it is considered the bible for any serious cellist. There is no such thing as an accomplished cellist who has not treated Popper as a religion at one time or another. Channing Robbins was my cello teacher for the first two years at Juilliard, and he was so passionate about the cello that his love for the instrument eclipsed his love for music itself. He knew the 40 Popper etudes like the back of his hand, and he once said the entire spectrum of cello playing was covered in nine of the most difficult etudes. Now I had another new goal, which was to master those nine etudes which I had previously studied, but had never worked up to a high level. Specifically, I began working on etudes 18 and 21, and the benefits were numerous. Etude 18 is three pages of fast notes played single bow and etude 21 is two pages of running notes, played eighteen notes to a bow. These two studies demand intricate coordination skills that are extremely difficult, and practicing them on a daily basis proved even more therapeutic for my hands than physical therapy could have been. As I began gaining proficiency with these etudes, it was clear my brain was actually finding new pathways to the muscles because each day my hands were becoming more responsive to the commands from my brain.

I distinctly remember the first of two physical therapy sessions that took place at my home during the lowest point in September, 1999. They were dedicated solely to regaining the use of my fingers. The therapist was creative and she came up with a great idea. She had me work with my miniature chess set that I had previously used for studying Bobby Fischer's games. I had almost no control over the muscles in my fingers, and it was a formidable challenge to insert the tiny pegs on the bottom of the chess pieces into the small holes in the center of each square of the board. At first it seemed impossible, but with daily practice I began getting the pegs in the holes. She also told me that playing the piano as well as the cello, would be a great form of therapy for the hands and fingers. The auditions were doing a great job of providing some needed motivation, and getting serious about regaining my foundation on the cello was proving to be a wise investment in many respects. It was exciting because I was actually reliving a time almost twenty-five years earlier when nothing else in my life mattered but learning to play the cello.

After several months of intense practicing every night until 3:00 – 4:00 am, time was running out to get ready for the L.A. audition. It was obvious I would need at least another year to be ready, but I boarded the plane and took the audition anyway. The audition did not go well at all, and it was an absolute disaster in many respects. The first item to complicate matters was when I was greeted by a member of the L.A. Philharmonic who escorted me on to the stage then sat several feet away while I played the audition material behind the screen (a screen is a large curtain used to assure a musician's anonymity during auditions). It was just my luck this person happened to be a woman I dated for one year while we were students at Juilliard. I began to play the Haydn D Major Cello Concerto and every note sounded like a struggle. All I could think while trying to play was that my former girlfriend, who had no idea what I had been through, must have been thinking what a washed up loser I was after such a short time in Philadelphia. I was so nervous that both hands were trembling and it was impossible to keep the bow from shaking. After the Haydn concerto the audition committee asked for the cello solo from Beethoven's opera *Fidelio*, and it went just as badly, if not worse. After just a few bars, I heard those dreaded but expected words from the audition committee behind the screen, "Thank you!" I walked off the stage with no pretense of advancing to the next round. Because of all the time and effort that went into preparing for this audition, I stuck around to hear the official announcement that I had been cut.

Diane Allencraig, a terrific flutist (or flautist) who previously had a one-year position with the Philadelphia Orchestra lived in Los Angeles, and she and her husband graciously extended an invitation for me to stay in their home during the time of the audition. After I was eliminated, I offered to babysit their young son Alex so the two of them could have a date night out. When they returned from their night out they were worried because the house was dark and quiet. I had fallen asleep reading to Alex and we were both down for the count. Preparing for the audition on top of fighting MS and running a full-time schedule of playing in the orchestra and teaching, left me totally exhausted and I'm pretty sure it was young Alex who put me to sleep. The next day Diane and young Alex took me to Disneyland, probably with the hope of improving my spirits after losing an audition. The audition debacle was heavy on my mind the entire time, but I remember getting some fresh pineapple on a stick from one of the vendors in the park. It is impossible to explain, but that blossom in the desert remains with me today as the best part of the audition and one of the most delicious things my taste buds have ever known.

The flight home from L.A. provided ample time to reflect on the postmortem of the audition, but more importantly I realized that it was not a total loss and some real progress had actually been achieved. I may have been busy licking my wounds from a bad showing at the audition, but there was much to be happy about. There had not been a single word from MS in two years, the lost physical strength was returning, my cello playing was making a slow but sure comeback, and I had just taken a very tough audition. The bottom line was I had set a goal that may have been unrealistically high, but a great deal of time and energy was devoted to it and the benefits were immeasurable. I had not given up or given in to MS, and I was already thinking about what I could do to improve at the next principal cello audition. It was time for a pat on the back for someone who could have easily and realistically opted for permanent disability.

One particular bright spot from that audition happened on the flight home on United Airlines. This took place several weeks after 9/11 and it seemed the entire nation was afraid to board an aircraft. United was eager to get people back flying again, so I took advantage of their promotional round trip flight from Philadelphia to Los Angeles for 15,000 miles. I booked two round-trip tickets (one for the cello and the other for yours truly) for 30,000 miles, and the flight to L.A. went without a hitch. On the return flight an overzealous flight attendant had my cello in her crosshairs, and she relentlessly harassed me about it. Prior to takeoff she insisted the cello go in a storage cabin on board the aircraft. I showed her the ticket for the seat that had been purchased for the cello, but she was determined to not let up. She looked at the ticket with a frown and insisted I put the cello in the seat upside down. I explained this position would subject the instrument to damage, and she walked away with a sour face. Then she returned with the pilot who assessed the situation but decided to allow the cello to remain in the seat.

Upon returning home, I immediately wrote a letter to United Airlines describing the embarrassing situation in front of everyone on the aircraft, and the utter humiliation while "flying the friendly skies." While a round trip airfare of 15,000 miles may have been a cheap date, I politely demanded a full refund of the miles used to purchase the seat for the cello. Lo and behold, several weeks later I received a letter from United apologizing for my ordeal and they credited 15,000 miles to my account for the seat for the cello. It is often said that money won is twice as sweet as money earned, and this one was sweet indeed as my cello ended up flying for free.

Ironing out my Nerves

Before moving on to any more auditions, the issue of nerves had to be resolved, so problem solving in this case was best done quickly and efficiently by getting to the root of the problem. In previous auditions I normally had nerves of steel, but the MS had also taken its toll on my confidence along with everything else. I can remember being nervous performing, but I had never had a previous experience where my hands were shaking to the point it was interfering with my playing. The chemical option of taking Inderal was not realistic as that would only have been a bandage that would not have addressed the core issue. The obvious solution to regaining confidence suddenly dawned on me, and it happened to be something that would provide unforeseen benefits as well. People will become skilled at something they do on a regular basis, so if I was serious about getting my nerves under control while playing for people, I had to constantly play in front of people. Playing in the cello section of an orchestra provides plenty of cover as there are many other cellists playing the same part, and it does not present a challenge for the nerves. Playing solo cello for people is a very different story, but playing solo cello at an audition is the most stressful experience one can imagine.

I called up nursing homes in my area and began playing for their residents on a regular basis, as often as twice each week. The employees of the nursing homes were thrilled to have a professional cellist volunteer to play for the residents, but the residents loved it even more. After several months of playing at nursing homes several times a week, the fear and self-consciousness while playing in front of people began to abate, and I truly enjoyed seeing what a difference I was making in the lives of people who tend to feel they are no longer able to contribute to society. I was once told you should go to bed each night having done something to make someone's day better, so if playing the cello for residents of a nursing home isn't going to make someone's day better, I don't know what will.

It was here I found a chance to once again raise the bar and set another higher goal, so I chose to learn and perform the Suite No. 6 in D Major for solo cello by Johann Sebastian Bach. I had never studied this work and I had previously shied away from it for a good reason. It is a seven movement monster originally written for a cello with five strings, which makes playing it on a four string cello extremely difficult. Attempting this work on the cello is as difficult as wrestling with a grizzly bear, so I began devoting several hours of patient work to the suite each day. It would be more than a year before it was ready to be played in front of anyone, so in the meantime the nursing home residents would have to be satisfied hearing the other Bach suites.

Another opportunity to raise the bar was seized during my visits to the nursing homes, and that was the chance to actually perform the etudes by David Popper. It is one thing to study these etudes, but it is another thing to perform them for people. When performing on unaccompanied cello, you are totally naked because there is no piano or any other instrument to provide cover or support in any way, and performing Popper etudes is a true test of cello skills. While Popper etudes may be a test of cello skills, I have always believed that playing unaccompanied Bach is the true test of a musician. Performing both the Popper and Bach on a regular basis worked wonders for the nervousness issue and it took only a few short months before it was back under control. As for Popper and Bach on solo cello - if you can make it there, you can make it anywhere.

The Detroit Symphony Principal Cello Audition

The next audition on the list was for the Principal Cello position of the Detroit Symphony. Once again I spent a great deal of time and effort preparing for the audition, but things were different this time. It was one year after the disastrous L.A. Audition, and there were several things going in the right direction. The use of my hands was actually beginning to return to normal, my cello playing was coming back, and after a year of playing in nursing homes I was completely regaining control of my nerves under pressure. After flying into Detroit and stepping outside of the airport, I was struck by a blast of arctic air. It was late fall, not even winter yet, it was bitterly cold outside, and I remember thinking how miserable I would be living in this climate. I picked up my rental car, drove to the hotel near the hall, checked in and began meditating to get complete mental control for the audition the following day. At the audition the nervousness was present, but my hands were not shaking and I played at a far more respectable level than I had at the L.A. Philharmonic audition. I did not pass the semi-final round but felt successful because I played an audition of difficult material and did not embarrass myself.

The Baltimore Symphony Orchestra Principal Cello Audition

The Baltimore Symphony Orchestra Principal Cello audition repertoire list included the 18th etude from *The High School of Cello Playing* by David Popper. This is one of the most difficult of the 40 etudes in the book, and by coincidence this is the one I was using to regain the use of my hands and fingers. I was constantly practicing this etude backstage and during the breaks of the Philadelphia Orchestra rehearsals, so when it appeared on the BSO audition list, my colleagues in the cello section somehow thought the audition was fixed for me. Nothing could have been further from the truth because I did not even pass the semi-final round of this audition.

Regardless, the aftermath of the audition left a surprisingly good feeling because I had not embarrassed myself and I even felt somewhat proud of my showing. During the audition my nerves were under control to the point my hands were not shaking, but I remember my shirt being completely soaked with sweat the entire time. Despite not passing the semi-final round in any of the three auditions, there would be no losing hope. I was actively taking major symphony orchestra principal cello auditions instead of being on permanent disability. Anytime I felt down about the audition results, all I had to do was step back and reflect on Dr. Sergott's prognosis.

The Philadelphia Orchestra Associate Principal Cello Audition

The Philadelphia Orchestra Associate Principal Cello position was the last audition I took and it was particularly tough because it meant playing for my colleagues in the Philadelphia Orchestra. When you play solo in front of your colleagues there are generally two outcomes: if you play well you are billed a strong player, and if you play badly you are branded a lousy player. With that hanging over my head it was impossible to do anything close to my best. After playing the difficult prelude to that sixth Bach suite which flopped, I played the first movement of the Lalo Cello Concerto, which went fairly well because by that time I had settled in. Next on the audition was a list of solos from the orchestral repertoire, and I actually felt good about the way they went. In top-flight auditions there is no room for someone who needs time to settle in; I was eliminated after the first round.

This was my last audition and even though I wanted to be the Lance Armstrong of the cello after conquering a major illness, I did not come close to winning a single audition. Alas, there is little to be ashamed of. When Dr.

Markowitz said I did the impossible, I can safely say I've landed among the stars.

Self-pity

As part of the recovery plan following the vicious third attack, I began volunteering time more than I had ever done previously. My volunteer work actually took on a life of its own with school visits, fund-raising events for the Philadelphia Orchestra and playing the cello for a variety of good causes such as retirement communities, nursing homes and schools. At one point I was visiting a different school each week and visits to nursing homes and retirement communities were often taking place as often twice a week. I even organized two annual Habitat for Humanity days in Camden, NJ, and participants included musicians, staff and board members of the Philadelphia Orchestra. During the time this was taking place, I wondered what was driving all this volunteer work because there were moments I honestly wondered if I was just acting the part. As time progressed and my health began improving with a vengeance, the unforeseen benefits of the volunteer work turned out to be far greater than I could have imagined. The reason behind this motivation remained a mystery until one day in a Philadelphia Orchestra rehearsal when I was hit by a sudden revelation that clearly explained everything. Without any realization I had begun devoting time to volunteer work to eliminate any possibility of self-pity.

It is common knowledge that women who suffer from depression have been known to snap out of the depression after giving birth. A likely explanation for this is the new and unprecedented purpose in life, when a newborn requires the mother's complete attention. This makes sense because the need to procreate is written into the human program, and along with that need is the necessity to care for a newborn. If this was not written into the program, the survival of the human race would likely be in jeopardy. As I began devoting time to improving the lives of those less fortunate and in far more need, I was drawn away from worrying about my own situation and focused on helping and serving others. One needs only to look at dogs for a deeper understanding of self-pity, because dogs have none. A dog that suffers from a deformity or the loss of a limb will not become depressed over its predicament because it is too busy enjoying the simple pleasures in life.

As time progressed it was clear the volunteer work had produced substantive benefits for my mind and body, so it was once again time to raise the bar and establish a new and higher goal for placing the needs of others before myself. This time it would not be the needs of other people – it would be the needs of the environment. Devoting time and energy to green living would serve to keep my mind focused on the positive, and less time and energy would be left for dwelling on the losing hand of cards I had been dealt. My new goal consisted of several environmentally friendly projects and one eco-hobby in particular.

Chapter 29

Environmentally Friendly Living

"Be kind to the earth. It's not Uranus." - Unknown

The laughter from seeing this bumper sticker nearly caused me to drive off the road, but the fact is environmentally friendly living leads to healthy living. An environmentally friendly diet is far healthier than one that is synthesized in a laboratory. A healthy diet will better enable the body to work in harmony with the mind. Several environmentally friendly projects I undertook were lifestyle changers, and the first was to begin composting food scraps rather than continue a lifelong habit of disposing of them in the trash. Food scraps from vegetable matter are the key ingredients of a compost bin, whereas scraps from an animal-based diet such as meat, fat and bones have no place there. One immediate and noticeable benefit from the absence of discarded food scraps was the elimination of any garbage odor in the kitchen. Food scraps make up a large portion of the trash produced in the U.S., so I also dramatically reduced my weekly contribution to the more than 1,600 landfills in this country.

Minimizing Energy Usage

Every species adapts to its surrounding environment, but humans are the only species that adapt the surrounding environment to their needs and desires.

Channing Robbins, my cello teacher at Juilliard who owned a summer home in Connecticut, once told of his practice of opening all the windows in his house at night, then rising at 5:00 am to close each one and draw down the shades. Trapping the cool nighttime summer air in a house will prolong and often negate the need for air conditioning. It is amazing how a simple helpful hint from someone can remain with you and shape your values and actions for the rest of your life. Several years later in 1985, I purchased my first home and followed Channing's advice. It was no surprise when I was rewarded with bragging rights to the lowest summer utility bills on the block. Unless it was an oppressively hot night, the open windows lowered the house temperature to the low 60s. This kept the house cool and comfortable until the late afternoon when the air conditioning switched on for the first time in the day. To this day, I continue this practice and it has become even more effective in my current home, which has solid concrete walls on the lower floors. Solid concrete walls efficiently retain heat and cold, In fact, they actually mimic the thermodynamics of a cave that remains at a constant temperature year round. Not only did Channing's story of his Connecticut house remain with me, it inspired me to look for other obvious ways to adapt to my surrounding environment.

The Environmentally Friendly Lawn

The first summer following the purchase of my house in 2001 saw a severe drought which resulted in restrictions on lawn watering and car washing. Every lawn in my neighborhood looked like it was dying of thirst except for my neighbor's lawn directly across the street. His front yard looked like a beautifully manicured golf course, totally void of weeds or dead spots. One day I went over for a neighborly chat to find out if he was guilty of midnight watering, and his response was puzzling:

"Nope, I don't water it."

"You don't?" I asked.

"Nope. And I don't feed it or use any weed killers either." He replied.

When asked how this was possible, he revealed his lawn was zoysia grass. It was amazing because this invasive species not only looks great in the summer, but it has a thick and tenacious root system that will choke out anything that even resembles a weed. The thought of owning a house with a nice looking lawn without the use of herbicides, pesticides, fertilizers and potable water, always remained something of a fantasy – until now! My neighbor gladly let me trim his overgrown lawn that had methodically annexed much of his sidewalk and driveway, and these trimmings were then planted around my lawn about one foot apart. Within a few years I had the same perfect looking lawn, without the use of herbicides, pesticides, fertilizer or potable water. When my house was sold in 2010, saying goodbye to the lawn was a bitter pill to swallow because I had given it so much time and energy. The buyer inherited a beautifully manicured lawn with little appreciation for the effort.

The Veggie Diesel – An Eco-Hobby

In 2007 my former high school music theory teacher Steve Zvengrowski gave me his diesel powered 1984 Volkswagen Quantum station wagon with only 134,000 miles on the odometer. Volkswagen diesels have a reputation for longevity and for logging many more miles than a comparable gasoline engine. I was fascinated with this car because it was designed with the express purpose of fuel efficiency, and its tiny fuel sipping four-cylinder engine got an incredible 50 miles to the gallon. Steve purchased this car new in 1984 and kept it in excellent condition, so this was the opportunity to fulfill my biggest eco-fantasy – to run a diesel car on waste vegetable oil. I had read about people who were doing this, and it was an exciting concept. After flying down to Steve's home in North Carolina to pick up the car, I drove it back to South Jersey and got busy making plans for the conversion. Soon I would no longer be on my knees serving the oil companies.

The first step was to contact Greasecar, the main company that sells the conversion kit, which is a simple system that converts older diesel vehicles to run on waste vegetable oil (WVO). This is how a diesel engine runs on WVO:

No modifications are made to the diesel engine, the diesel injection pump or the injectors. The car becomes a dual fuel vehicle. The conversion kit includes a second fuel tank which is mounted in the spare tire well of the car, leaving the existing diesel fuel tank in place and unmodified. The newly installed WVO tank has an internal heat-exchanging coil that scavenges hot coolant from the engine to heat the WVO. When heated, the viscosity thins and the hot reused cooking oil functions identically to diesel fuel. When cold, the engine must be started on straight diesel fuel, and when the thermostat detects the temperature of the coolant to be 180 degrees Fahrenheit, it opens and hot engine coolant is circulated to the radiator to keep the engine from overheating. With a WVO system, the driver then flips a switch that changes the fuel from diesel to heated WVO. The car then runs flawlessly on WVO, but two minutes before shutting down the engine, the WVO is purged from the fuel system by flipping the switch and changing the fuel supply back to diesel fuel, which ensures the next cold startup. The humorous part of driving a car that runs on WVO is the odor emitted from the tailpipe, typically reminiscent of whatever was last cooked in the oil.

My lucky source for an unlimited supply of filthy WVO was a local Japanese restaurant, which conveniently provided the greasy stuff in its original five-gallon cans. This high quality soybean oil was used primarily to make tempura, so the exhaust from the car had an odor that was a cross between tempura and French fries. People were often bewildered by the concept of a car that runs on WVO, and everyone thought I was getting a great deal by not paying for fuel.

Operating a vehicle on WVO is a major undertaking and it is by no means free. The waste oil had to be picked up at the dumpster of the restaurant and placed in the back of the car. When transporting this dirty oil home, every bump in the road seemed to cause the oil to celebrate by splashing the inside of the car. After arriving home with the messy stuff, I poured it into a barrel, enabling the impurities to settle to the bottom. I ran the cleaner WVO on top (which is still dirty) through a filter system so the impurities in the WVO would not clog the diesel injectors. The entire process of preparing and filtering WVO would have been a good feature on the television show: *Dirty Jobs*.

After filtering the lighter WVO, the bottom of the barrel was left with a heavy sludge that I scooped out and disposed of. I tried composting the gooey substance but it overwhelmed the compost bin, so it sadly became part of my contribution to America's landfills. Once filtered, I poured the WVO into the five-gallon gas cans that went along for the ride on long trips. Getting the filtered WVO into the gas cans without spilling it was an endless challenge. The floor of my garage often looked like an aerial view of the Gulf of Mexico after the infamous Macondo blowout. Filling the WVO tank from the five-gallon gas cans was another messy project, and I often spilled the gooey slimy stuff in the back of the car.

After two and a half years of driving around on WVO, the car's low coolant sensor unknowingly failed and a coolant hose coincidently burst while I was on the highway. I had no idea the engine had overheated from running without coolant for 20 minutes at highway speed, and the resulting heat produced a crack in the cylinder head. Finding a replacement cylinder head for a 26-year-old diesel car for a reasonable price proved impossible, so I sold the car as is, along with the entire WVO system. Even though I had not paid for diesel fuel for two and a half years and 30,000 miles, there had been some major expenses with the project. The cost of the WVO conversion kit, the filtering system, the filters and the time invested had far eclipsed any fuel savings. Running a car on WVO was a great experience, and I was sad to see it come to an end. It consumed a great deal of time, energy and resources, but it made me realize there is something to be said for the convenience of handing the automotive refueling engineer a credit card and saying, "Fill 'er up."

MS, on the other hand, was a plight that I was not so sad to see come to an end. From my first symptoms in December 1998 to my lowest point, I went from a state of denial to a state of shock to a state of hopelessness. From this state of hopelessness I moved forward to a state of sheer determination. It was as if I was experiencing the five stages of grief, only not in order. I rejected acceptance first and I put anger to its best use. Every experience in my life was used to develop a battle plan that would be used to combat an incurable disease. Having any chance of being successful required a new level of discipline and determination. Everything about my life would now be focused on crafting an organized and systematic approach to beating MS. I gained a great deal of knowledge from researching, studying and embracing the will of those who accomplished the impossible. These were people who displayed superhuman physical, mental and artistic skills. My entire life would then be devoted to becoming one of them.

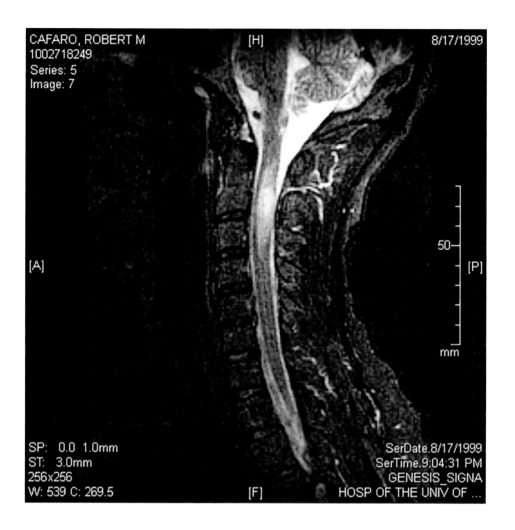

MRI Showing 3.5 cm lesion in spinal cord.

August 17, 1999

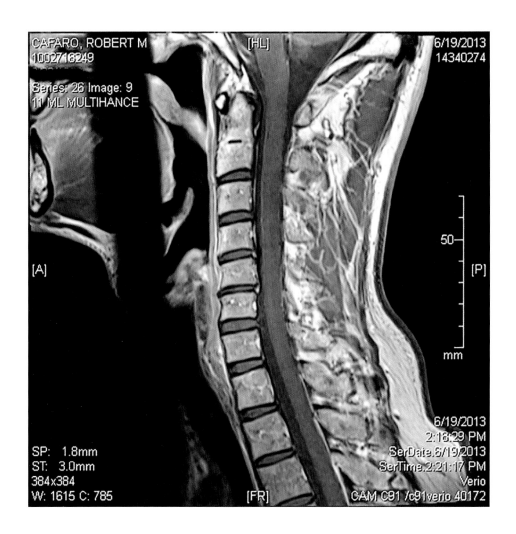

MRI Showing 3.5 cm lesion in spinal cord gone.

June 19, 2013

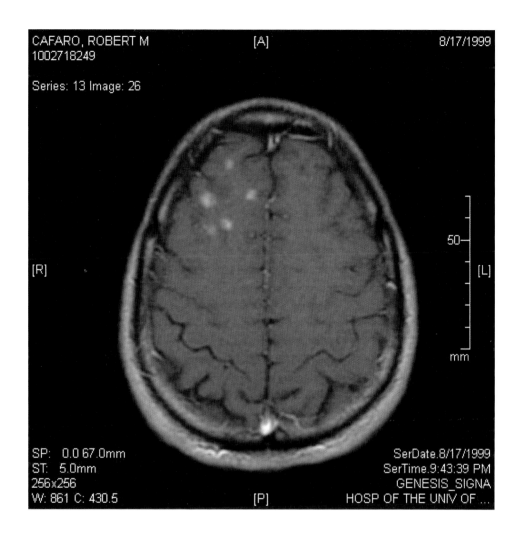

MRI Showing multiple lesions in the brain.

August 17, 1999

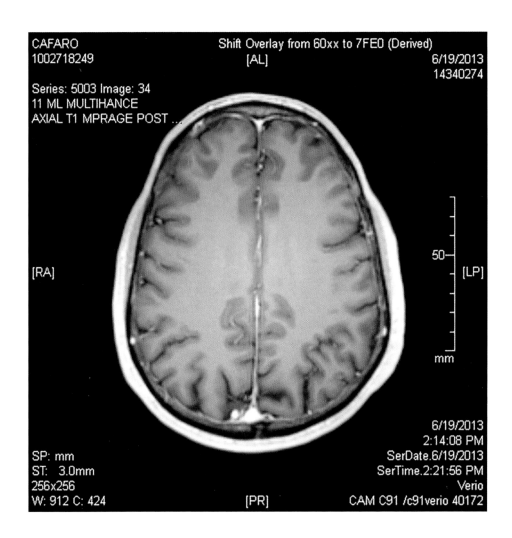

MRI Showing multiple lesions in the brain gone.

June 19, 2013

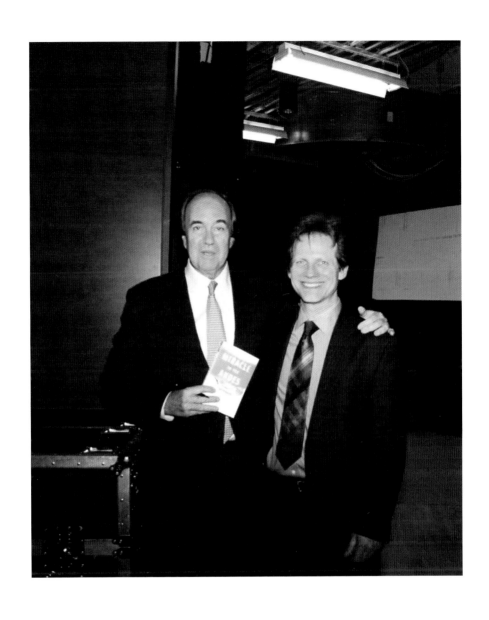

Bob and his hero, Nando Parrado,
Survivor, and Author of *Miracle in the Andes*
April 15, 2013

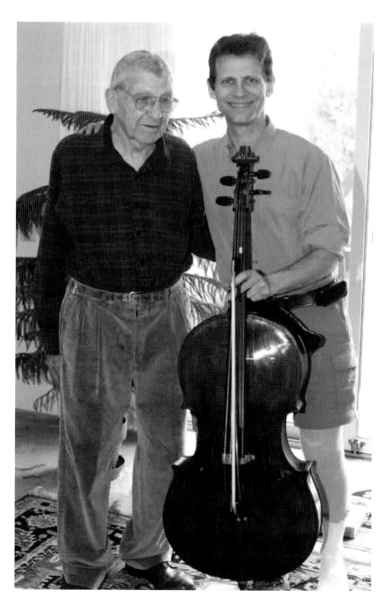

Bob and his spiritual guide, Bill Golz,
with the 'Ex-Golz' Santagiuliana Cello from 1816, Venice
May 10, 2012

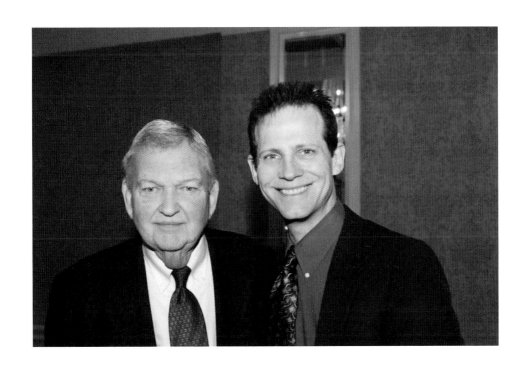

Bob and his mentor and teacher, the late Bill Stokking,

Former Principal Cellist of The Philadelphia Orchestra

May 7, 2007

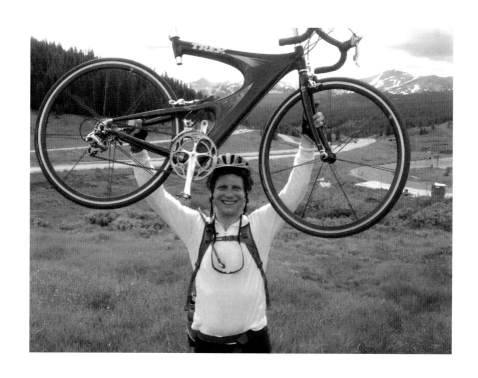

Bob, after reaching the summit of Vail Pass – Colorado
July 11, 2011

"Out of difficulties come miracles" - *Jean de la Bruyere*

-Part II-

Chapter 30

How I Beat MS – Step-by-Step

"The role of the physician is to entertain his patient while nature takes its course."

- Voltaire

For many people this will likely be the most important part of the book. Previous sections may be useful and at times entertaining, but I needed a step-by-step process when I was diagnosed and had nowhere to turn.

I took several important steps in my war against MS. In a perfect world, those steps would work for everyone – but this is anything but a perfect world. Regardless of what health challenge one faces, it is important not to be complacent by leaving everything to the doctor or medicine. Much of what it takes to beat any serious illness will come from within.

This section will provide details of my diet, exercise regimen and meditation. In order for them to be effective, they must be practiced with the following:

- A willingness to make the necessary sacrifices of lifestyle
- The mindset to stay focused and disciplined
- The commitment and perseverance to devote unlimited time and energy, and to never give up

Diet – Energy from the Sun

All life energy comes from the sun, and the most efficient way of getting that energy to the body is with vegetable matter. Meat is a complete food for the body but it contains impurities that can lead to health problems, and it is an indirect way of getting the sun's energy to the body. The human diet is omnivorous yet we only consume the meat of animals that are herbivores. Therefore, it is best to go directly to the source for food that is best for the fight against MS - that food is plant matter.

At the time I began researching a diet for MS, the one good book I found that seriously addressed a diet for MS patients was *The MS Diet Book* by Dr. Roy Swank. His recommended diet is well thought out and researched, but I took it one step further by going even more basic. The diet I finally adopted was customized for my body and tailored to battling MS.

Here is a list of the books from which my diet was crafted:

- The *Okinawa Program* by Bradley J. Wilcox, M.D., Craig Wilcox, PhD., and Makoto Suzuki, M.D.
- *Nolan Ryan's Pitcher's Bible* by Nolan Ryan and Tom House
- *The MS Diet Book* by Dr. Roy Swank
- *The Complete Illustrated Book of Yoga* by Swami Vishnudevananda

After a great deal of research and thought, I began living exclusively on carefully selected foods. These foods on my list are all worthy of consideration, but similar to any exercise or meditation program, the best diet is the one that is customized to the needs of each individual. I based my food selections on the basic needs of the human body. These foods are pure and unadulterated - human body fuel in its natural state. Some people have mild or severe allergies to seeds, soy, nuts, salmon, certain fruits or vegetables, so planning a diet for an individual should be approached with caution. Any food that may cause an allergic reaction should be strictly avoided.

"We are all born in nature. Most people spend their lives walking away from it. When we get sick, then it is time to run back!"

- 'Mustang' Bill Wasylenco, Owner - Mustang Stables - Bensalem, PA.

One of the most valuable lessons learned during my experience battling MS is that many common illnesses are inflammatory responses to questionable but accepted modern dietary practices. The human body was not meant to withstand the onslaught of today's toxic lifestyle, and the word toxic refers to alcohol and tobacco as well as the ingestion of modern foods and drinks that are designed in a laboratory and mass produced as inexpensively as possible. Processed and fried foods that are high in fat, salt and sugar, synthetic sweeteners, artificial colors, flavors and preservatives, are the seedbed for many common ailments, yet society is largely resistant to making any change back to a simple diet.

One theory identifies modern refrigeration as a major contributing factor to our decline in health, and it makes good sense. Along with the convenience of the refrigerator comes an increase in meat and dairy consumption. This is reflected in the rise of heart and arterial diseases. Another theory involves the Betty Crocker Cookbook, which first appeared on the scene in 1950. This cookbook is heavy on vegetable shortening which is highly processed, and the theory links this cookbook with a sudden rise in heart disease as well as a reduced lifespan. Vegetable shortening became popular back then because it was a mainstay in many of the cookbook's recipes, and that ingredient is hydrogenated vegetable oil, which is a foreign substance for the human body.

The human body is highly resilient to toxins to a point, and this is where quantity is the key. The parts-per-million scale is used by agencies from the EPA (Environmental Protection Agency) to OSHA (Occupational Safety and Health Administration), and this is a subject worth considering. In his film, *Super Size Me*, Morgan Sperlock illustrates the consequences of a diet based solely on fast food. At the conclusion of that 30-day experiment, he gained a substantial amount of weight, he became ill in many ways, and his doctor said he was "pickling his liver." The human body can handle small amounts of many toxins – provided they are indeed small amounts.

The first of my lifestyle changes focused on diet, and a major factor in my success against MS was the adoption of one simple and original dietary rule: **If you have to read the label, don't eat it.** I also abstain from foods and drinks that could affect the central nervous system. This includes caffeinated drinks -such as coffee, energy drinks and tea- but herbal teas are permitted. Omitting caffeine is my own personal theory and there is no evidence to back it up. I have also eliminated carbonated drinks. Carbonation is an acquired taste; it is a rare occurrence in nature. The only liquid I drink is water and I make it a point to drink plenty. I also put spicy food under the microscope when searching for answers to MS. Once again, this is my own personal theory; many will disagree with my opinion that spicy food adversely affects the central nervous system. For me, the idea originated from what my body has communicated to my brain.

When a person consumes extremely spicy food, it often produces changes to the body that are visible to others. This can be observed when people indulge in such food, and the unnatural result is coughing and watering eyes. It is also common to see people sweating profusely from eating extremely spicy foods, and that could be a possible sign of the body's attempt to cool down what it senses is an overheated system. Another basic reason I avoid spices in my food is that food with spices tastes far better, so I tend to eat more. It is highly doubtful I am the only person with that weakness, but a major tactic in my battle plan was to reduce caloric intake, and that obviously successful plan continues to work.

Water

Early in my recovery when I was fortunate to have discovered the Water Cure, I began drinking 64 ounces of filtered water every morning before any food. This proved to be a wise investment, as it immediately helped improve my horrible state of health and it was instrumental in ridding my body of all the toxins that were present in my system. Over a period of eight months I was pumped full of intravenous and oral steroids, naproxen, ibuprofen, acetaminophen, antibiotics, gadolinium (MRI contrast dye) and interferon (Avonex®). The interferon injections and the accompanying side effects continued for another four years, but the Water Cure cleansed my body and successfully softened the blow of the side effects.

Drinking a large amount of water first thing in the morning is at the top of my recommended list because it resulted in a fast improvement from my lowest point, and it continues to work well as a preventive measure. After seeing my MRIs from 2013 that were physical proof of a complete recovery, I have scaled back my morning water intake to only one liter (33.81ounces) before any food. Drinking 64 ounces of water in the morning is somewhat radical and it is not always practical, so I am now content to start each day with just a single liter.

My list of foods does not address the size of the portions because I make it a point to stop eating when I am no longer hungry. When I follow this practice, eating should be complete after only a few bites. Eating slowly and chewing well is also important because the stomach needs time to communicate a message of satisfaction to the brain. That deer in Shenandoah National Park spent much of the day foraging on small amounts of raw food, and probably never experienced the sensation of a full stomach.

Sunflower Seeds

Sunflower seeds are one of my favorite foods and they just happen to be nearly perfect for the body. I choose only organically grown sunflower seeds that are raw, unsalted and not roasted. When sunflower seeds are dry roasted, the natural oil inside the seed is cooked and the seed is modified from its natural state. If sunflower seeds are roasted in oil, the changes go even further as the additional cooked oil adds excess calories for the body to deal with. The most commonly found sunflower seeds in stores are roasted in oil and salted, which places it in the category of processed food. That brings us back to the three things that are rare in nature but abundant in today's diet – salt, fat and sugar.

The human body needs a surprisingly small amount of sodium. When foods with added salt are consumed the basic sodium requirement is exceeded and the body is challenged with the task of expelling the excess. This unnecessary problem is difficult for the body to handle and I believe excess salt wreaks havoc in many ways. An overdose of sodium is very common in our modern diet, and the human body has ways of cleverly responding with a variety of warning signals. Unfortunately, these warning signals are often hidden by medications of today that successfully mask the signals. Some of these medications will actually produce new and different warning signals of their own. Hence it is best to deal with basics by reducing the amount of salt in the diet. One other major benefit from eating raw sunflower seeds as a snack is the total void of sugar. "Bacteria love sugar" is a famous saying, and bacteria are the known seedbed for tooth decay. Hence, it is wise to learn the discipline of enjoying just plain sunflower seeds as a preferred snack.

Sunflower seeds are beneficial because they contain selenium, which is a proven cancer fighter. They also contain magnesium and copper, which keep bones strong. In addition, they contain vitamin E, which is great for the skin, and antioxidants, which are known to reduce inflammation. Each day after drinking my morning water, I address my first sign of hunger with a few handfuls of plain organic sunflower seeds. There is no sure way of knowing how much this helped my fight with MS, but this amazing food has a place at the top of my recommended list because my results are difficult to dispute.

Sunflower seeds contain vitamin E, copper, vitamin B1, manganese, selenium, phosphorus, magnesium, vitamin B6, folate, vitamin B3 and polyunsaturated oil.

Raisins

Raisins and sunflower seeds work together to make a highly nutritious snack that rivals the taste of an energy bar. Energy bars are often heavily processed with unwelcome ingredients, so I opt for the mix of sunflower seeds and raisins, which is pure and far superior. Conventional raisins are often high in pesticides and preservatives, so choose only organic raisins. Dried fruit that is refrigerated in a sealed container will remain fresh for a long time, so it is always a great idea to have raisins and sunflower seeds on hand as emergency food. Society constantly tempts us with unhealthy food when we are on the run and lack the time to get quality food, so keeping sunflower seeds and raisins in a day pack or purse at all times is the perfect solution. Enjoying healthy food is possible after the taste buds relearn to enjoy food in its natural state. As a society our taste buds have been conditioned with high amounts of salt, fat and sugar, therefore food in its natural state will initially have a bland taste.

Raisins contain fiber and protein plus the minerals potassium, manganese, copper, iron, phosphorus, magnesium, thiamin, riboflavin, niacin and vitamins B6, C and K.

Nuts

There is limitless information available on how nuts do everything from helping to avoid and fight cancer, to extending one's lifespan. Nuts are also a great source of protein, which is doubly important for anyone avoiding meat and dairy. Early in my recovery, nuts became a main part of my diet and they remain so today.

Nuts are great because they contain the good monounsaturated and polyunsaturated fats, omega-3 fatty acids, fiber, vitamin E, plant sterols and L-arginine.

Almonds

Research pointed out the many benefits of eating almonds so they became the majority of nuts in my diet, and once again I chose raw and organic whenever possible. Unfortunately my dietary practice consisted of eating them by the handful, and a subsequent price was paid for chewing too many at one time. The chewing of multiple almonds caused hairline fractures in four of my molars, and three of those molars eventually succumbed to the fractures and failed. When a tooth fails, it must be ground down and capped, so I am now the proud owner of three crowns. A crown on a tooth does not make one feel like a king, but it is nice to be able to chew normally. It is often said that a smart person learns from his mistakes, and a brilliant person learns from the mistakes of others. Therefore, my advice is to exercise brilliance by eating almonds one at a time and chewing slowly.

The benefits of almonds include protein, calcium, magnesium, potassium, niacin, vitamin E, fiber and riboflavin.

Pistachios

Pistachios taste great alone, but when they are added to sunflower seeds and raisins, the taste competes with the best energy bars on the market. When you combine the naturally occurring fat in pistachios with the natural sugar in raisins and the consistency of chewed sunflower seeds, the high salt content in energy bars will not be missed. Growing up, I remember pistachio nuts that were most often loaded with salt and colored red, but now it is easy to find unadulterated pistachio nuts without the salt and red food dye.

Pistachios are a good source of monounsaturated fatty acids and they are high in fiber, protein, copper, manganese, phosphorus, magnesium, vitamin B6 and folate.

Blueberries

The credit for my discovery of blueberries to fight MS belongs to Dr. Markowitz. When I asked him about foods that would be helpful in fighting MS, he mentioned blueberries because they contain a chemical that benefits the brain. I have a great deal of respect for Dr. Markowitz for his constant desire to learn and his willingness to think beyond traditional medical schooling. At every one of my appointments, he eagerly shared his latest knowledge that he gained while being on the lookout for ways to help his patients.

Organic or Conventional?

An analysis of pesticides in produce by the not-for-profit Environmental Working Group (EWG), is based on the results of 43,000 tests for pesticides on produce that were collected by the U.S. Department of Agriculture and the U.S. Food and Drug Administration between 2000 and 2005. On a scale from 1 to 100, with one being the best and 100 being the worst, blueberries are rated 25th on the list of tested pesticides, which I reluctantly found to be acceptable. Organic blueberries can be difficult to find, and when they are available, they are often prohibitively expensive. Another concern was my new life of living alone, and along with weekly spousal and child support payments, there was the constant worry of making ends meet. On my road back to health I consumed large amounts of blueberries, therefore conventionally grown blueberries is one of the few areas where I bent the rules. Each spring there is always a bumper crop of locally grown blueberries in Southern New Jersey, so that is when I stock up.

Fresh blueberries along with other fresh berries have a short shelf life, so when the magic of dehydration was discovered I bought spring blueberries in bulk and ran my two dehydrators around the clock. My dehydrators are 9-tray models made by Excalibur, and each unit has the capacity to dehydrate 15 square feet of food. A dehydrator uses a relatively small amount of energy because it is nothing more than a simple heating coil with a fan that circulates the warm dry air. One of these units uses slightly more electricity than a 100-watt incandescent light bulb, so in winter the dehydrator doubles as a heat source in the house. In the summer, I place it outside so there is no competing with the air conditioner. Dehydrated fruit and vegetables contain almost no moisture, and sealed they will last for years in the freezer. A bag of dehydrated blueberries is another excellent food to keep handy throughout the day.

Blueberries have more antioxidants that any other fruit or vegetable tested to date. Antioxidants are known to strengthen the immune system, so this is a no-brainer.

Other Berries

Blueberries are not the only berries that are great for health. I also eat strawberries, raspberries, blackberries and cranberries. Berries are difficult to grow without pesticides, so I make it a point to choose organically grown berries when it is possible as well as practical. The above-mentioned berries also dehydrate and store well. Since my days of recovery, I have made it a practice to eat berries by themselves as a meal or a snack.

Blueberries, strawberries, blackberries, raspberries and cranberries are good sources for anthocyanins, antioxidants, catechins (flavonols that support the antioxidant defense system), dietary fiber, ellagic acid, fiber, gallic acid, ORAC (oxygen radical absorbance capacity), phytochemicals, quercetin, rutin, salicylic acid and vitamin C.

Apples

During my recovery, apples were a mainstay in my diet and they remain so today. My favorite apples are Gala, Fuji, Honeycrisp and Red Delicious. Organic apples have become so common today that they are even available at Costco and BJ's Wholesale Club, so I always opt for organic.

Apples are a good source of vitamin C, B-complex vitamins (riboflavin, thiamin and vitamin B6), fiber, phytonutrients, and the minerals calcium, potassium and phosphorus. In addition to all of the good in apples, they contain almost no fat, sodium or cholesterol.

Bananas

Once bananas are ripe, they can be placed in the refrigerator where they will remain in that ripe state for almost two weeks. Do not be fooled by the blackening of the peel over the two weeks because the inside of the banana remains delicious. Bananas are also one of the very best fruits for dehydrating. Dried bananas are one of my main foods on the overseas orchestra tours because they do not need refrigeration. Bananas are considered one of nature's perfect foods for good reason; when a baby's very first food is a mashed up banana, it should be considered food for thought.

Bananas are a good source of vitamin B6, vitamin C, potassium, magnesium, iron and copper.

Pineapples

Pineapples are one more fruit that was a big part of my diet during my recovery. They are normally not ripe when on the grocery store shelf, but they ripen nicely in a few days out on the kitchen counter. Ripeness is evident by a sweet fragrance and when the leaves can be easily pulled from the top. The pineapple can then be refrigerated until it is ready to be cut. Once cut, the chunks or slices will remain fresh in a sealed container for a good amount of time. Pineapple slices also work exceptionally well in a dehydrator. The dried slices are one of my favorite overseas tour foods.

Pineapple is an excellent source of vitamin C and it is the only known source of the enzyme bromelain, which is believed to have many benefits including reducing inflammation. Pineapple also has vitamin A, calcium, thiamin, riboflavin, vitamin B6, folate, pantothenic acid, magnesium, manganese, potassium, antioxidants and polyphenols such as beta-carotene.

Grapes

Green and red grapes are both part of my diet, but I always choose organic grapes because of the pesticides that are often used to grow conventional grapes.

Grapes are rich in vitamins C and K, and they are an excellent source of antioxidants.

Avocados

During the first few years of my recovery, I totally avoided all wheat and gluten. I do have a weak spot for sandwiches, so avoiding wheat and still enjoying a good sandwich was possible with rice bread made by Food for Life®. I gave up dairy and mayonnaise along with wheat. The perfect sandwich spread turned out to be a ripe avocado. The avocado may be a complete and satisfying food by itself, but in a sandwich with other delicious ingredients, it is superior to standard spreads such as mayonnaise. At one point, I tried Nayonnaise, a tofu-based mayonnaise substitute that was tasty, but it had too many ingredients for my restricted MS diet.

Avocados are a great source of protein, vitamin B6 and folic acid, and they contain vitamin E, glutathione and monounsaturated fat.

Wild Alaskan Salmon

I avoid farm-raised salmon because most farmed-raised fish are raised in overcrowded, unsanitary conditions and they are given antibiotics as a preventive measure. If that is not enough, farm-raised salmon are commonly fed food dye for a brighter and more appetizing appearance at the dinner table. Salmon is an excellent food for the body, but wild salmon should be the first choice. Wild salmon is amazingly beneficial for the central nervous system, so each year I took advantage of the summer runs of wild Alaskan salmon and stocked up my freezer.

I prepare wild salmon with basil, pepper and fresh ginger, and then it is cooked on the grill at a low heat but not directly over a burner. This turns the grill into a low-heat convection of sorts, because the salmon is not cooked directly over the heat source. Baking salmon in the oven is also great. I cook it at a temperature of about 200 degrees Fahrenheit, and only until it begins to ooze out the sides. Overcooking wild salmon should be avoided because it destroys the valuable nutrients and negates the nutritional benefits. Dehydrating wild salmon works well, but a major drawback is the need to refrigerate the dried salmon. Fish oil cannot be dehydrated, and unrefrigerated fish oil at room temperature will quickly become rancid. Hence, this is not one of my touring foods.

Wild salmon is high in vitamin B12, vitamin D, selenium, vitamin B3, omega-3 fats, protein, phosphorus, vitamin B6, iodine, choline, pantothenic acid, biotin and potassium.

Recipe for Wild Salmon (grilled or baked)

- Wash and scale the salmon.
- Generously place thinly sliced ginger on top of the salmon.
- Sprinkle with pepper and basil.
- Bake in the oven at 200 degrees Fahrenheit for 15-20 minutes to ensure it is not overcooked or dried out.

Another option is to cook the salmon on the grill.

- On the grill, place the salmon on an area that is not directly over the flame. At a low heat, cook the salmon only until it begins oozing out of the sides.

Watercress

During childhood, I developed a fascination with watercress after reading the short story, *The Doctor's Heroism*, by Villiers De L'Isle-Adam. This is a story of a very sick and frail man who is seen by a doctor and he is diagnosed with a terminal illness. The doctor informs him there is no available treatment and he only has several months to live. Since there is no hope for the man the doctor asks if he has money, and the man just happens to be wealthy. The doctor then experiments on the man by telling him his only hope is to go to a warm climate and live on nothing but watercress for six months. The man then leaves the office and the doctor has no expectation of ever seeing him again. After six months of following the doctor's advice of living on watercress, the man returns to the office in such a remarkable state of perfect health that the doctor does not recognize him. After the man reminds the doctor that he is the patient with the terminal illness who was sent to the warm climate to live on watercress, the doctor immediately takes a pistol out of his desk drawer and shoots the man in the head, killing him instantly. When the police arrive to make an arrest, they find the doctor examining the man's organs with a magnifying glass in search of answers to the man's mysterious and complete recovery.

That story left a powerful impression on my young mind, and it stayed with me to become an important part of my recovery from MS thirty years later. During my recovery, I did not actually live on a six-month diet of only watercress, but raw watercress did become one of the main foods in my diet. It may seem like fantasy to think watercress could have such amazing healing power, but if the mind believes watercress has that power, then it is entirely possible. Once again, consider the unexplained placebo effect in many clinical trials.

In 1985, I was a member of the Baltimore Symphony for one season before leaving to join the Philadelphia Orchestra. I always missed the musicians in Baltimore after having such a great time with so many people, and many of the friendships I made then have continued to this day. Before departing for Philadelphia, several people in the Baltimore Symphony asked if I would ever consider returning one day as their principal cellist, and that question perpetually occupied a space in my mind. My time in Baltimore may have been limited, but I loved the city and surrounding area as much as the symphony.

When I was first hired, I rented a room in a house north of the city right near a bike shop. One day I stopped in just to have a look. This was in 1985 when the mountain bike craze was in its infancy, and I ended up buying my first mountain bike. The thrill of going off road on a bicycle was a novelty and I spent plenty of time on the bike trails around the two reservoirs north of the city. The Loch Raven and the Pretty Boy reservoirs are the water supply for the city of Baltimore and they are magnificent bodies of water in pristine condition with no swimming allowed and no surrounding development. At night several of the musicians and I would often sneak into areas of the reservoirs at the places only the locals knew, and we would go swimming. I was twenty-five, and I felt like a wild carefree teenager once again.

One of the other wonderful memories near the two reservoirs was the natural spring water that came from the ground, and once again, only the locals knew of this. The source of this water was at the side of a spring located well north of the city, and I managed to find it from only a description and verbal directions. The taste of this spring water was amazing so I brought along five-gallon jugs on every visit. The water flow at the source was quite slow and filling the containers was time consuming, so I sat there in a meditative state in the beautiful surroundings while the jugs filled.

One time I happened to notice an abundant and familiar looking plant that was growing wild in the spring, and upon closer examination, it looked exactly like watercress. I plucked a piece out of the spring and had a small taste, and was shocked it was not just watercress – it was the strongest tasting, freshest watercress one could ever experience. My eyes followed the stream, and for as far as they could see, the bank was completely overgrown with this magic vegetable. I retrieved a large shopping bag from the car and promptly filled it with this miraculous gift of nature. On the drive home, I enjoyed munching on bite after bite of my latest discovery. Unfortunately, the euphoria was short lived as gastrointestinal issues arose from consuming a large quantity of fresh watercress. It was such a shocking novelty to my digestive system, that it somehow perceived the watercress to be a potent laxative rather than a vegetable.

Watercress has so many benefits that a Center for Disease Control (CDC) study labeled it, "the most nutrient-dense food," and it is at the top of the list for "powerhouse fruits and vegetables."

Brown rice

Brown rice is one of two grains that comprised a large part of my diet during my recovery. If uncooked and kept in the refrigerator brown rice will last a very long time. Cooked brown rice does not freeze well, but it will last nicely in the refrigerator in a sealed container.

Brown rice is high in selenium, manganese, naturally occurring healthy oils, anti-oxidants and fiber.

Quinoa

I generally alternate between two grains - brown rice and quinoa. Considerable debate exists on exactly what quinoa is. Some define it as a grain and others define it as a seed but either way it does not contain gluten, which is important to anyone on a gluten-free diet. If it is a grain, quinoa is the only one that contains protein, which is important for those who avoid meat and dairy. I eat quinoa along with steamed vegetables and tempeh or tofu. In my case, I practiced discipline by eating it straight with no sauces, oils or spices. If one is serious about beating MS or any other serious illness, it is important to remember: Eat to live; do not live to eat.

Quinoa is a true wonder-food as it contains all nine of the essential amino acids. It is also high in anti-inflammatory phytonutrients, making it an important weapon when fighting autoimmune diseases.

Soy Beans

Soybeans cooked and added to rice or quinoa were also a regular part of my diet. Once again, I only choose organic soybeans. Unless soybeans are organic, they are most likely GMO (genetically modified organism), and I have not researched the GMO issue enough to give an opinion. The fact is GMO food is a recent introduction into our food chain and too little is known about any risks, particularly when one has a weakened or compromised immune system. Therefore I avoid GMO foods whenever possible.

Soybeans are good sources of copper, manganese, phosphorus, protein, iron, omega-3 fats, fiber, vitamin B2, magnesium, vitamin K and potassium.

Tofu

I always enjoyed tofu so there was no discipline involved in eating this. Tofu is one of those chameleon-like foods that readily adapts to almost any dish or flavor. Tofu by itself is rather bland and tasteless, but it has a unique ability to absorb and enhance the flavor of anything to which it is added. While tofu is admittedly a processed food, the processing formula has been around for more than 2,000 years. It is still considered an extremely healthy food.

Tofu is high in protein, iron and calcium and since it is made from soybeans, it contains many of the same benefits.

Tempeh

Tempeh is partially fermented soybeans made into a cake, then cut into small sizes. Tempeh is up there on my list of favorite foods because it can assume the taste of many spices and flavorings, and the texture resembles that of meat. It is made from soybeans therefore it is high in protein and has all the same benefits as soybeans. One advantage of the partial fermentation process of tempeh is the neutralization of the gaseous properties of soybeans.

Trail Mix

Trail mixes are generally delicious, but 'Go Take a Hike' is by far the best trail mix I have ever tasted. It is rather expensive but every ingredient is organic and it is well worth the cost. The way I cut costs on this one is by ordering in bulk directly from International Harvest, the distributor in Mount Vernon, NY. My one reservation about this tasty food is the large amount of natural sugar in the dried fruits as well as the carbohydrates. After I discovered this magic mix, I noticed an increase in the size of my waist, and a belly that was beginning to hang over my belt. Since the belly was not paying rent, I have cut back significantly on the consumption of this trail mix and have subsequently limited my intake to one or two handfuls per day.

Go Take a Hike trail mix contains organic raw ingredients including goji berries, mulberries, golden raisins, cacao nibs, cashews and pistachios. This trail mix is a good source of fiber, vitamin A, vitamin C and iron, but it is high in calories, carbohydrates and natural sugars, so I would strongly advise eating only small amounts.

Sweet Potatoes or Yams

Sweet potatoes are an easy meal to prepare. After they are scrubbed, poked with numerous holes and placed in a Pyrex dish, they are baked in the oven at 350 degrees Fahrenheit with a convection fan (if equipped). Bake for up to two hours, but only until they are soft and begin to caramelize. Once cooled, they can be wrapped and placed in the freezer where they will assume a long life. A medium sized sweet potato from the freezer will thaw and be ready to eat in a few hours, and this constitutes a healthy and unprocessed substantive meal by itself.

Sweet potatoes or yams are rich in fiber, vitamin A and vitamin C. They also contain smaller amounts of potassium, calcium and iron.

Sushi

The varying MS rates on the planet may seem mysterious, but I am convinced the reason has more to do with lifestyle than anything else. One statistic in my research that stood out was the lower rates of MS in Japan. I have been to Japan numerous times and this country, which is located on the other side of the planet, has a population that is nearly half that of the United States. Japan makes good use of space to enable 127.3 million people to live in an area that is equal in size to the state of Wyoming. How does Japan with its serious overcrowding and environmental issues have MS rates that are much lower than the U.S.?

Considering lifestyle, the traditional Japanese diet is largely rice and vegetables, with much smaller amounts of fish and meat. If our modern processed fast food and meat diet is new to the West, consider how much newer it is in the East. Another difference with the Japanese diet is the quantity of food consumed in the average meal. America is home of the "all you can eat" culture, and Japan, and Okinawa in particular, is more of the "eat what you need" culture.

Avoiding restaurants was definitely helpful during my fight against MS, but there were many times when this was not realistic. I do enjoy sushi, therefore it became one of my restaurant favorites. When eating sushi, wasabi is not part of my meal due to its extreme spiciness. I omit soy sauce because of the high sodium content. If one chooses to eat sushi without the traditional wasabi and soy sauce, it had better be fresh because old, raw fish makes for a rather unpleasant dining experience.

For those who doubt my theory behind Japan's lower rates of MS, consider the traditional Japanese diet, the custom of smaller portions and a markedly reduced amount of processed food. Ironically, as the Japanese increasingly acquire a taste for Western meat and fast food, they are experiencing a rise in the rates of ailments more commonly associated with the West such as obesity and diabetes.

Sushi is select cuts of mainly raw fish; therefore, the benefits of eating fish are even greater because the nutrients are not cooked. There is valid concern about the risks of consuming raw fish, but I have yet to experience an illness from bad sushi. The nose and taste buds make good sentinels for fish that should not be eaten. If the sushi has an unpleasant smell or taste, do not eat it and send it back.

Fresh fish is a low-fat food that is high in quality protein. It is rich with omega-3 fatty acids and vitamin D and vitamin B2 (riboflavin). It is also high in calcium and phosphorus, and it is rich in minerals such as iron, zinc, iodine, magnesium and potassium.

Split Pea Soup

This is one of my classic meals, and one that I frequently prepared with a hot plate and backpacking pots in five-star hotel rooms on the orchestra tours. Food prepared in such a setting must be good "transit" food with a hardy shelf life; therefore, dried split peas and soy sauce fit the bill perfectly. The orchestra has a strict policy of not allowing any food in our wardrobe trunks on the tours, so I made clear to the orchestra staff a necessity to bring my own food and they were great about it. On tours, the vegetables included in this dish were the ones available locally. The recipe is a simple one.

- Organic split peas
- Onions
- Celery
- Carrots
- Other available fresh vegetables
- Soy sauce – use low sodium organic soy sauce sparingly

Soak the peas overnight in a ratio of two cups water to one cup split peas. Overnight soaking will effectively address any gaseous issues with the peas.

Bring the peas to a boil, then lower heat to simmer.

Add the sliced or chopped onions. (I created this dish using a small cutting board and hotplate in a five-star hotel room on the orchestra tours, so I was not very selective about the specific cut of an onion.)

Add the vegetables later so overcooking does not compromise the nutrients.

Add pepper and a minimal amount of soy sauce to taste.

Dried peas, split and cooked, are high in molybdenum, fiber, manganese, copper, protein, folate, vitamin B1, phosphorus, pantothenic acid and potassium.

Steamed Vegetables

Steamed leafy vegetables are better than baked or stir-fried vegetables because light steaming leaves valuable nutrients intact. If plain steamed vegetables seem boring and unappetizing, adding fresh sliced ginger to the steaming process adds a tasty dimension to the steamed vegetables. I strongly advise learning the discipline of foregoing rich taste by training the taste buds to appreciate food in its natural state - without salt, fat and sugar. My favorite vegetables for steaming are watercress, green, red or rainbow chard, kale and collard greens. Adding tempeh or tofu to the steaming mix further enhances the flavor, and the addition of a grain such as brown rice or quinoa makes a complete and healthy meal.

Ginger for Energy

One of the big challenges from my third MS attack was my lack of strength and stamina. This presented challenges during the orchestra rehearsals and concerts, and I would lose my mental focus and begin to doze right in my chair. My first step to address this issue was to start sitting on the edge of the chair when playing the cello, without the comfort of leaning back. That helped somewhat, but it did not solve the problem.

One of my worst experiences happened at an orchestra rehearsal during a summer at the Mann Music Center in Philadelphia. The rehearsal was being test videoed and displayed on a giant screen over the stage. The Mann Music Center is an outdoor venue, and the purpose of the screen is to enlarge the orchestra for the audience to see up close. During the rehearsal, I was struggling to stay awake, and after losing the fight, I began to snooze. Suddenly my stand partner nudged me with his bow and I opened my eyes to see all my colleagues laughing at me. The cameraman was so amused by a Philadelphia Orchestra cellist sleeping during a rehearsal that he was unable to resist the temptation of a narcoleptic close-up on the giant screen. How embarrassing!

After that humiliating experience, I was determined to find a way to stay awake on the stage without the use of medication. The solution to this issue was a simple one – dehydrated ginger. A slice of dehydrated ginger has an extremely potent taste, and placed under the tongue it will keep anyone from dozing off. Carrying around fresh ginger is not realistic, but carrying around dehydrated ginger was perfect because of its total lack of moisture. Peeling fresh ginger may be time consuming, but having fresh ginger on hand makes it well worth the effort. When hot water is added to crushed, dehydrated ginger, it makes a phenomenal cup of energy-rich tea. Chopped fresh ginger that is crushed with a garlic press also makes great ginger tea.

Ginger has been used worldwide for thousands of years to treat many ailments including calming the stomach and aiding with digestion. It is considered one of those miracle foods with many healing properties. My use of ginger is generally for the purpose of providing energy and staying awake.

Sautéed Vegetables

During my recovery, sautéed vegetables became one of my staple foods; this remains true today. When my children were young, they loved going to the local "All You Can Eat" buffet, and there I always made a beeline for the Mongolian barbecue station to assemble a mix of vegetables for sautéing. The mix consisted of onions, Chinese cabbage, broccoli, bean sprouts, and whatever was available among the vegetables of the day. At a Mongolian barbecue your selected vegetables are handed to the chef, who normally sautés the mix in oil and sugary spicy sauces. I always exercised discipline, and insisted on having mine sautéed with only water. At first, it was an admittedly bland taste that left much to be desired, but over time my taste buds acclimated to the natural taste without the addition of salt, fat, sugar and spices.

Sandwiches

Sandwiches are a great part of the diet to fight MS, so here are a few sandwich ideas that work well:

Tempeh Veggie Sandwich

- 2 slices of Food for Life® bread
- Ripe avocado used as a spread
- Fresh or dehydrated tomato slices
- Sliced tempeh (has the texture of meat)
- Sprouts
- Sliced cucumber
- Fresh watercress or other available spring mix greens

Wild Alaskan Salmon Salad Sandwich

- 2 slices Food for Life® bread
- Wild Alaskan salmon mixed with ripe avocado instead of mayonnaise
- Fresh or dehydrated tomato slices
- Fresh watercress or spring mix greens

Portion Size

The subject of food quantity is just as important as food quality. The subjects in *The Okinawa Centenarian Study* not only ate good quality food, but they stopped eating when they were 80 percent full. Overeating is one of the unhealthiest things for the human body, so cancelling your membership in America's all-you-can-eat club is strongly advised. After my third attack, I experimented with how little food my body would need, and there was a benefit to learning to be hungry much of the time. Cutting caloric intake lengthens the lifespans of mice, rats, rabbits and fruit flies, and human beings are no different. Reducing caloric intake will be a difficult discipline for most people, but it is important to consider exactly how far one must go to beat a disease like MS.

There is no proof and only theories of what causes MS. When one is diagnosed with the disease, it is important to consider what will help and what will make it worse. My mind kept going back to that deer in Shenandoah

National Park, and that was instrumental in helping to decide what foods would be avoided.

Foods That Were Strictly Avoided

I conceived my diet from a combination of research, fear, trial and error. With my central nervous system in such a frail state, the decision was made to avoid any food or drink that could possibly affect the central nervous system. The following is a list of foods I avoid:

Caffeine

I eliminated caffeine because it is a stimulant, which means it stimulates the central nervous system. Luckily, I never got started with coffee because I never acquired a taste for it. Give an infant a sip of fine roasted Columbian black coffee, and he will spit it out and scream. Many people are addicted to coffee to the point they get a headache without their daily cup. That should be taken into consideration when deciding to give up coffee. In addition, all caffeinated tea and energy drinks should be avoided.

Alcohol

Some people believe alcohol is actually good for the body, but I find it difficult to concur due to the origin of the word 'intoxicated'. I am a firm believer that alcohol in any amount is toxic, but it is possible there may be some benefit when it comes to countering any arterial buildup that is caused by the unhealthy fats found in fatty and fast food.

Processed food

Modern processed food was eliminated because my goal was to give up the affluent Western diet and live on a diet commonly associated with poorer nations that have low rates of MS. Today's processed food may not be directly linked to higher rates of MS, but that was a chance I was not willing to take.

Fried food

When food is fried, the caloric content increases many times over. The caloric content of the cooked oil alone eclipses the caloric content of any food before it is fried. The body must then deal with digesting the oil that was used in the frying process. Fried food was completely ruled out of my diet and that included Japanese tempura, despite being lightly fried in higher quality soybean oil.

Dairy

All dairy was ruled out including milk and milk products, such as cheese and yogurt. We live in a society that is highly influenced by the dairy industry. From the time we begin to read and watch television, we are targeted by ads that say it is unhealthy to avoid dairy products. We are the only species that drinks another species' milk; therefore, I believe there may be something inherently unnatural about it. Modern refrigeration has made it possible to consume ever-larger quantities of meat and dairy. This has resulted in a generally unbalanced Western diet. Most of my diet consists of food in its natural state, most of which does not require refrigeration.

Salt, Sugar and Flour

There is a Russian saying: "Salt is the white poison and sugar is the sweet poison." I was once told we should not eat anything that is white, and this means salt, sugar, and white flour. This made good sense, so out they went.

Eggs

Even though Dr. Hoffman believes one or two eggs per week is beneficial, I was not willing to take any chances. *The MS Diet Book* by Dr. Roy Swank had me frightened of them; therefore, eggs were off the table. However, since my total recovery I have resumed eating an occasional egg, but not more than one or two per week.

Meat

I rarely ate meat before the days of MS, and when I did, it was only to be polite in certain social settings. After my third attack, I became deadly serious and disciplined about everything, and I stopped eating meat under all circumstances. In 1985 when I won the Philadelphia Orchestra cello audition, the Executive Director of the orchestra required the newly hired members to get a complete physical examination. When the doctor who administered the exam saw the results of my blood work, he was astonished to see my cholesterol level at a low 115. At that time, I was playing in the Baltimore Symphony and living alone. My simple diet consisted of mostly raw food and watercress, and I was fasting one day each week. One day I intend to get back to that discipline of a weekly fast because it was a very clean way to live. I hope that doing so is a proactive move and not a reactive move that is triggered by another health crisis.

Two Restaurants I Frequent and Recommend

There are two restaurants I frequent on a fairly regular basis. One is in Philadelphia, PA and the other is in Saratoga, NY.

Essene

Essene is a serious health food store and café located at the intersection of Bainbridge Street and 4th Street in Philadelphia. It is one of the best health food stores in the area. Their café consists of a large buffet that offers many excellent choices. In February of 2000 when I first became single and lived alone, my cooking skills were quite limited. Shortly after that solitary part of my life began, I happened to be in Essene and I struck up a conversation with David Goodrick who was Essene's head cook at the time. He had heard that I was a cellist with the Philadelphia Orchestra, and he wanted to know if I gave cello lessons. His inquisition caught my attention because I give cello lessons, but I also get hungry sometimes. I broached the possibility of giving cello lessons in exchange for cooking lessons. David was thrilled with the idea of giving cooking lessons, but his lessons turned out to be different than what I had envisioned. He instructed me to come to Essene with my own set of knives and be ready to learn how to cook.

David Goodrick is not only an excellent chef; he is also a demanding teacher. On my first available free day I showed up at Essene ready to cook, and the lessons began. They turned out to be more like basic training in the military than basic cooking lessons. Wasting no time with small talk, he handed me an apron from the bin. We then went downstairs to the giant walk-in refrigerator and he loaded my arms with the ingredients for several dishes, one of which involved baked mushrooms. The plan was to make enough to feed 40 people, so David handed me a gigantic box of mushrooms. We proceeded back up to the kitchen where I was given instructions to wash the entire box of mushrooms. Utilizing the only system I knew to wash mushrooms, I turned the cold faucet on to a trickle and began methodically thumbing the first mushroom clean. With a stern look and a raised voice of impatience, David made it clear that this was no way to wash mushrooms. He filled the large sink halfway with water then dumped the entire box into the drink. He then vigorously swirled the mushrooms around in the water and they were quickly and efficiently cleaned by this patented method. The job of washing ten pounds of mushrooms that would have taken several hours doing it my way was condensed into just a few minutes.

The lesson continued when I began slicing the mushrooms. David watched over my shoulder and, thankfully, was highly critical of my technique. I was cutting with the knife in my right hand while holding the vegetables in my left hand with straightened fingers. A slip of the knife while holding the vegetables this way could easily have had ended the career of any professional cellist! David promptly grabbed the knife from my hand and demonstrated the proper way of holding food while it is being cut. You hold the food with your fingertips curled underneath while resting your knuckles on the side of the blade. With this technique it is much more difficult to add a fingertip to the recipe while simultaneously ending your career as a professional cellist. This basic rule of safety seems so obvious now but it was anything but obvious at the time. Needless to say I was much more skilled in the kitchen after David's basic training than I was before I met him.

Avoidance of restaurants during my recovery stemmed from the fear of not knowing what was in the food or how it was prepared. My "lessons" with David Goodrick at Essene continued for several months and during that time it was reassuring to see that only carefully selected, healthy ingredients were used in the food served at Essene. Unlike the corporate world of Wall Street, the health and well-being of Essene's customers is more important than company profits. Since that time in the kitchen, my first-hand experience has enabled me to feel comfortable and confident dining at Essene. One of the greatest things about this restaurant is its practice of offering salt-free dishes. The buffet offers two completely salt-free items that I gravitate toward when filling my plate. The only bad thing about the café at Essene is the deliciousness of the food. This tempts one to eat far more than necessary. The Okinawa Centenarian Study subjects stopped eating when they were 80% full, but when I eat at Essene it is such a treat and the food is so good, that I tend to keep eating even when I am 100% full!

Four Seasons Health Food Store and Café

I first discovered Four Seasons Health Food Store and Café early in my tenure with the Philadelphia Orchestra. Going to Saratoga, NY for three weeks every summer is truly one of my favorite parts of playing in that great orchestra. Four Seasons has grown in popularity to the point where it has recently expanded the café to meet an ever-increasing demand for its food. In addition to the bigger café, Four Seasons' health food store has moved to a bigger location nearby.

My first time in Saratoga was in August of 1975 when I was student at the School of Orchestra Studies. I have been to many beautiful places on the planet and Saratoga is one of my favorites; it is where I hope to one day settle down for good. The Philadelphia Orchestra has been the resident orchestra at the Saratoga Performing Arts Center since its opening in 1966, and every August since 1985 I have spent three happy weeks there. To this day, missing the orchestra's 1999 Saratoga season haunts me, but the viciousness of my third attack offered no choice in the matter.

I first discovered Four Seasons when I was walking around downtown Saratoga. At the time it was on a much smaller scale than Essene in Philadelphia, but the food has always been excellent and healthy! When I speak to the people that work at Essene and Four Seasons, I always make it a point to congratulate them for choosing a profession that makes the world a better place to live. When my assessment of their livelihood is met with skepticism, I explain how they do not work for a collection agency, nor are they denying valid health insurance claims for a living. Instead, their job helps people achieve and maintain a better quality of life. As a bonus, they happen provide food that is not only extremely healthy, but extremely pleasing to the palate as well! Four Seasons' buffet is on a somewhat smaller scale than Essene, but their menu changes daily and it usually varies twice a day.

Every spring I volunteer one week in March to visit schools in the Saratoga region. The purpose for these visits is to promote the Philadelphia Orchestra's three-week summer season in August. The trip in March is always hectic because the schedule consists of three one-hour visits to three different schools a day, for five days straight. One joyous pleasure during this week is getting to dine at the Four Seasons Cafe two times a day!

When my dream of living in Saratoga comes to fruition, my plan is to give back to the school music programs that did so much to change my life in 1975. I was lucky enough to begin studying the cello in public school in third grade; every child should have that same opportunity. The other part of my Saratoga plan is to work part-time at the Four Seasons Café and learn the preparation secrets behind their outstanding food.

When I die and go to heaven, I will know I am there because the Four Seasons' buffet will be the meal plan. I am currently still in negotiations with St. Peter regarding the matter, so I am not at liberty to comment on the progress of our talks at this time.

Chapter 31

Conditioning the Body and Training the Mind

The word coordination has a tendency to take on a new meaning when a person is diagnosed with MS, and that certainly held true in my case. I previously thought of coordination as only a skill of the body, but when the brain is not able to fully communicate with the muscles, it becomes an entirely new challenge of brainpower. Coordination is mind over muscle and coordination skills can range from the simplest tasks, such as pouring water into a glass, to such complex ones as playing the cello. Analyzing and applying a new approach to coordination was very helpful when it came to turning things around and relearning the use of my body. MS often attacks the ability of fine motor skills, and the effects can remain long after an attack. After my vicious attack during the summer of 1999, many of my coordination skills were stripped away to the point I was unable to write legibly or even hold a phone. Even playing the cello was no longer possible.

The daily practice of a few simple exercises was immeasurably helpful in rebuilding, maintaining and sharpening my coordination skills.

Juggling

I require that all my cello students learn how to juggle because it is a simple yet difficult hand-eye coordination skill. This circus trick does not demand muscle strength or stamina, and there is no chance of injury while practicing. I learned the basic juggling skills during my student days at Juilliard, but after my third attack, I brushed off the dust and began practicing juggling once again. This is an excellent physical therapy exercise for anyone fighting MS because it seems to force the brain to find pathways to control the muscles. Juggling will also challenge the aging process because reflexes and coordination tend to decline as we age. Keep in mind juggling is more a skill of the mind than a skill of the body.

Begin with three tennis balls or three small beanbags if you do not relish navigating around those tenacious dust bunnies that reside under the furniture every time you drop the ball.

Step 1 - The Basic Skill of Juggling with One Ball

Begin with one ball or beanbag. Start with your arms at your sides and your forearms pointing straight out with both palms facing up. Beginning with the right hand, throw the ball up to a level slightly higher than your head, and into the waiting left hand. Once the ball is caught with the left hand, reverse the process by throwing the ball from the left hand up to the same height and back into the right hand. Repeat the process going back and forth until a level of proficiency with both hands is achieved. Keep your eyes focused at the peak height of the ball's arc – do not let your eyes follow the ball. When practicing juggling, relax and try to move in slow motion, and only use the muscles that are necessary.

Step 2 - The Basic Skill of Juggling with Two Balls

This exercise begins with one ball or bean bag in each hand. Beginning with the right hand, throw the first ball slightly higher than your head and into the left hand. When the first ball is at eye level and before catching the first ball with the left hand, throw the second ball underneath the first ball – up to the same height and into the right hand. If performed correctly, the sound produced should be a lopsided "throw, throw – catch, catch." When a level of proficiency is achieved with this exercise, reverse and throw with the left hand first. Complete mastery of Step 2 is required before attempting Step 3.

Step 3 - The Basic Skill of Juggling with Three Balls

Start with two balls in the right hand and the third ball in the left hand. With the right hand, throw the first ball slightly higher than your head and into the left hand. Before catching the first ball with the left hand, throw the second ball under the first ball – up to the same height and into the right hand. Before catching the second ball with the right hand, throw the third ball up to the same height and into the left hand. Juggling three balls is a complete and continuous cycle that will be difficult and will take much practice. If the central nervous system is impaired in any way, extra patience will be required. I believe that if this skill is diligently practiced on a daily basis, it will implore the brain to find necessary pathways for communicating with and controlling the muscles. This is called neuroplasticity, which is a term I was unfamiliar with during my recovery.

Cycling

Riding a bicycle is an excellent way of maintaining coordination skills because the brain is multitasking by controlling many parts of the body simultaneously. It also sharpens reflexes by requiring the brain to make instant judgment calls for navigation and balance. After my third attack, I unexpectedly discovered it was still possible to balance on two wheels; I was on the bike several times each day to relearn and regain much of my lost coordination. This was instrumental in my recovery because cycling is an excellent workout for the body as well as the mind, and it served to rebuild my strength, stamina and confidence. There are many great balancing exercises but cycling is a complete exercise for the brain, body and cardiovascular system.

Become the Athlete

To beat MS or any other serious disease, the answer will not only come from a doctor or the latest FDA-approved drug. One must not only think like an athlete, one must become an athlete in every sense of the word. I am referring not to an ordinary athlete, but a top-level competitor who is in exceptional physical and mental condition. When a person is diagnosed with any serious illness, it is important to adopt the mindset of just such an athlete and remember the following:

- Battling this illness is a competition against a world-class opponent with an enviable winning record.
- No competitor wins every single match and no champion reigns forever – even MS.
- The fight against MS is much more than a competitive event. It is the fight for your life and it is one fight you do not want to lose.

- Studying and understanding the thinking process of the very best athletes is helpful because top-level athletes succeed in getting their bodies to achieve unbelievable feats.
- The best athletes live a disciplined lifestyle and they are highly self-motivated.
- One must be willing to sacrifice anything and everything that will impede success.

When fighting MS, one must make time to do what needs to be done; there can be no waiting for someone else to provide motivation. MS is an opponent that does not wait until you are ready to enter the ring, and it does not give a chance to regroup with one minute rests between rounds. This is a disease that fights mercilessly for 24 hours a day, seven days a week, and you must rise to the occasion with a total commitment to fighting back 24/7.

I followed my regimen for diet, exercise and meditation with discipline. That focused approach is a must for anyone who wants to beat MS or any other serious illness. It should be noted that disregarding a doctor's advice and stopping any prescribed medication is definitely not my recommendation. Neurology and medicine have made great progress in treating MS, and the available treatments should be viewed as vital weapons in the battle. It is important to consider my regimen only as an example of what worked for me to totally rid my body of MS. This mysterious disease affects each person differently, so the approach for each individual will be a unique and uncharted learning process.

My Exercise Regimen

MS Yoga

There are different types of yoga, so thought and consideration should be given to which form of yoga is best suited for those with MS. Hot Yoga, which has gained in popularity, is a form of yoga that is practiced in a studio where the room temperature is raised to over 100 degrees Fahrenheit. The theory behind hot yoga is to cleanse the body by sweating out toxins. My third attack struck right after strenuous long bike rides in extreme heat and humidity, therefore I believe practicing yoga in such an environment is risky and potentially harmful for those with MS. I strongly suggest practicing yoga in moderate or cool temperatures. Dr. Lublin reinforced this with his advice to avoid cardiovascular activity to the point of sweating. I totally disregarded his advice and subsequently paid a very heavy price with my third attack. During the first year of my recovery afterward, my house was kept at 60 degrees Fahrenheit in the winter, to keep my body from overheating and to fend off a dreaded fourth attack.

Preparing for Morning Yoga

After a night of restful sleep, slowly drink 32 to 34 ounces of filtered water to prepare for a morning session. When there is no longer any bloated sensation from the water, it is time to begin morning yoga followed by two 30-minute meditation sessions. Keep in mind the daily amount of water consumed should be one ounce of water for every two pounds of body weight. The human body and the blood in particular are mostly water, and the entire circulatory system is powered by water. The central nervous system depends on water for electrical conductivity, which is necessary for every bodily function.

The morning is the best time for yoga because the mind is rested, awake and most responsive. Food should not be eaten before morning exercise or meditation because blood will be diverted from the brain to the stomach for the purpose of digestion. My daily exercise routine always takes place before a morning shower and even before brushing my teeth.

Select a soothing quiet place for your session that has access to sunlight and is free of distractions such as a television or cell phone. The sun powers all life and even fossil fuels are stored sunlight, so there is a definite benefit to performing yoga exercises while absorbing energy from the sun. Distracting music should not be present during yoga or meditation, so the brain does not wander from focusing on the task.

During my morning yoga session, I listen to Glenn Gould playing the preludes and fugues from Johann Sebastian Bach's *The Well-Tempered Clavier*, because it is not of this world. It is impossible for me to accept that a human being actually composed such brilliant music, and I place Glenn Gould at the top of the list of Bach's interpreters. There is no doubt in my mind that if Bach had heard Glenn Gould play his keyboard works, he would have been very impressed. Bach is truly the voice of a higher being, and the spiritual experience of hearing Bach interpreted by Glenn Gould enhances my ability to elevate beyond the physical world to a world without physical limits. In that world, anything is possible – including beating incurable illnesses.

Yoga and meditation should be practiced first thing in the morning. If morning time is not convenient, learn the discipline of getting to sleep earlier in the evening so morning time is made available. Another reason for morning yoga is to free the body of the stiffness that results from lying motionless all night. Fresh oxygenated blood is the energy supply to the body, and it acts as an anesthetic for relief from the aches and pains that are brought on by several hours of sleep.

Step 1 - Breathing Exercises

Begin by sitting on the floor in a semi-lotus or cross-legged position, with the spine as straight as possible. I always sit slightly elevated on a pillow or cushion to keep the legs and feet slightly lower than the pelvis. If the position is uncomfortable sit with both legs to one side or simply sit in a chair. I lack the flexibility of a yoga master, so I gave up on the full lotus years ago. Even if one is unable to perform a full or semi-lotus pose, full benefits can be achieved by breathing deeply while sitting still and clearing the mind. In the semi-lotus position, I repeat a series of deep breathing exercises 5 – 10 times.

Proper inhalation is done in three stages:

- Using the diaphragm, inhale and completely fill the lower abdomen with air.
- Continue by filling the mid-abdomen.
- Lastly, fill the upper chest with air.

When the lower abdomen, mid-abdomen and upper chest are full, forcefully inhale three more short breaths without exhaling, then hold for a count of 10.

Proper exhalation is done in the reverse order:

- Empty the upper chest of air.
- Expel air from the mid-abdomen.
- Use the diaphragm to exhale all remaining air from the lower abdomen.

When all air has been exhaled, forcefully exhale three more times without inhaling, then hold for a count of 10.

Repeating this process several times produces a cardiovascular and aerobic benefit similar to running, but with far greater efficiency. The brain receives more blood than any organ in the body, and systematic breathing turbocharges the blood with oxygen to provide the brain with a morning awakening that is superior to caffeine. It also provides an infusion of energy that will later be used during meditation. It is normal to feel some initial lightheadedness, but with practice, the brain and body will grow accustomed to this new oxygen-infused blood flow.

Step 2 - The Cow Head Pose

The next step is to counter the semi-lotus or cross-legged position by assuming what is known as the cow head pose. In the cow head pose, the buttocks are on the floor and both feet are placed outside the upper legs. The toes then point outward and this provides both knees with a counter-stretch to the lotus pose. It may take several months to get comfortable with this pose and it may be difficult or impossible for some to ever achieve it, therefore it should not be considered mandatory. The cow head pose should be approached slowly and with extreme caution due to any risk of knee or ankle strain. Once in this position, I proceed to the shoulder exercises.

This next cross-elbow pose is part of the eagle pose. Place the right elbow inside the left elbow, and touch the nose with both hands. In this position, begin deep breathing exercises with five complete inhalations and exhalations. Then reverse the elbows by placing the left elbow inside the right elbow. Once again, touch the nose with both hands and perform five complete inhalations and exhalations.

This forward-stretching shoulder exercise is then countered by joining the fingers of both hands in the area of the upper back in the following manner: Place the right hand behind the lower back and reach up as high as possible – as if attempting to scratch a point on the upper back. With the left hand, reach back over the left shoulder and join the fingers of both hands. It could take months or it may be difficult or impossible for some to join the fingers of both hands, so patience should be practiced without the mindset of competitive yoga. What is right is that which is right for you. Even if the fingers do not meet up behind the back, hold the position at a point where it is comfortable and begin a series of five complete inhalations and exhalations. Then reverse the arms by reaching up the back with the left hand, and reaching back over the right shoulder with the right hand. Join the fingers or get them as close as possible, and begin a series of five complete inhalations and exhalations. When practicing the cow head pose and shoulder exercises, the point of discomfort should be the limit. If pain is felt, it means you have gone too far and you should ease up.

As the body ages, the joints, tendons, ligaments and meniscus tend to stiffen and cause chronic pain, so keeping them pliable becomes more important with each passing day. These daily exercises will help to delay the onset of arthritis, possible knee replacements and shoulder trouble, and they serve to ensure a better quality of life. Keep in mind an unhealthy diet and lack of exercise are welcome friends of the aging process.

Step 3 - The Spinal Twist

The importance of this exercise cannot be stressed enough. In 1999, there were at least 53 lesions in my brain, but an immense 3.5 cm lesion in the cervical region of my spinal cord caused my biggest problems. The spinal cord is the communication system used by the brain to control the entire body, so keeping the spinal cord limber will be beneficial for those with MS. The gentle stretching and twisting of the spinal cord will help get energy and fresh blood to where it is needed. Because the spinal cord is the system used by the brain to control the muscles, I recommend this pose as necessary maintenance for the body's communication system.

Sit on the floor in a cross-legged position, and place the right foot on the floor to the left of the left knee or thigh. Then place the upper left arm over the right side of the right upper leg; this prepares for the spinal twist to the right. With the right hand reaching far to the right side, touch the floor and twist the spine to the right to a point of comfort, and look to the right as far as possible. Hold this position while breathing deeply. With each exhalation, try to go deeper into the pose.

After 5 – 10 deep breaths, reverse the pose by starting from a cross-legged position, and place the left foot on the floor to the right of the right knee or thigh. Place the upper right arm over the left side of the left upper leg; this prepares for the reverse spinal twist to the left. With the left hand reaching far to the left side, touch the floor and twist the spine to the left to a point of comfort and look to the left as far as possible. Hold this position while breathing deeply. Once again, with each exhalation, try to go deeper into the pose. Continue to hold for 5 – 10 deep breaths.

There should be no pain felt when practicing this or any pose, but a good stretch should be felt in the back and the spinal cord. It has been many years, and I am only recently able to practice this pose with decent form. Even though my form is not perfect, I get it as close as possible while still reaping the maximum benefit for the spinal cord. Some people may find it difficult or even impossible to perform the Spinal Twist pose while seated on the floor. If that is the case, the benefits to the spine and back can still be achieved by practicing the pose while seated in a chair.

Step 4 - The Sun Salutation

The Sun Salutation is a well-known series of yoga poses I use to begin my morning session, but I have modified it specifically to fight MS. Instead of moving quickly through each pose, I assume each position and hold it for an extended period while breathing deeply.

1.   Mountain Pose

With good posture and a straight back, stand and face the sun if possible. Inhale deeply then exhale to experience the solid feeling of proper posture as well as balance.

2.   Upward Salute – Backward Bend

Raise the arms and hands straight above the head and shoulders, and begin bending backward slightly. In the beginning, bending back with the arms extended will be difficult, but with time and practice, it should become easier. Hold this position as far back as possible and inhale to capacity. Hold the breath, exhale and return to the standing position.

3.   Standing Forward Bend

Exhale and bend forward with the knees as straight as possible, and place both palms on the floor while placing the head between the knees. Unless one regularly practices yoga, this pose is easier said than done. I have been practicing yoga since my teen years, and I am still unable to do this pose without bending my knees. It is important to remember what is right is what you are able to do. Exhale as deeply as possible and with each exhalation, go deeper into the pose by bending farther forward and straightening the knees as much as possible.

4. High Lunge with Left Leg between Palms

From the standing forward bend position, extend the right leg straight back and place the right knee on the floor with the toes of the right foot curled up. The left knee should be over the left toes, and the left side of the chest is resting on the upper left leg. The left foot is between the hands, which are palms down, and flat on the floor. Extend and spread the fingers out while pointing the thumbs toward the toes. This daily stretch of the hands and fingers will help slow the aging process of the hands by working to keep the fingers and joints pliable. With the head up and while looking up, hold this position and breathe deeply. With each exhalation, relax deeper into the pose.

5. Plank Pose

Extend both legs and assume the raised position of a pushup, with only the toes and flat hands on the floor. In this position, breathe deeply but hold each breath in and out. Do not lock the elbows back, but instead bend them slightly to strengthen the arms and the upper body.

6. Forehead, Chest, Hands, Knees and Toes to Floor

In this pose, the toes should be curled upward with the knees touching the floor. Arch the back and point the butt up into the air. After the toes and knees are on the floor, the chest touches the floor with the stomach remaining off the floor. Tuck the chin down to the neck, similar to what one does when folding bed sheets, and place the forehead on the floor. In this pose, the only parts of the body that touch the floor are the forehead, chest, hands, knees and toes. Inhale and exhale deeply. With the chest extended out, the back arched and the butt up to the sky, deep breathing will take place naturally.

7. Cobra Pose

Lie flat on the stomach with the legs together and the toes extended out. Push on the floor to lift the body while keeping the legs and the hips on the floor. Bend up and back as far as possible, then hold and breathe. This pose is great for inhaling deeply because the entire abdomen and chest are extended out.

8. Downward-Facing Dog

This pose resembles the formation of a teepee because good form will place the body in the shape of that simple dwelling. Keep the palms out to the front and flat on the floor, with both legs back and both feet as flat on the floor as possible. Straighten the arms and legs, relax the shoulders and breathe deeply. With each exhalation, relax deeper into the pose. Keeping both feet flat on the floor with the knees straight, is very advanced. I am still unable to straighten my knees while practicing this pose.

9.   High Lunge with Right Leg between Palms

This is the reverse of pose No. 4. Extend the left leg straight back and place the left knee on the floor with the toes of the left foot curled upward. The right knee should be over the right toes and the right side of the chest is resting on the upper right leg. The right foot is between the hands, which are palms down and flat on the floor. Once again, extend and spread the fingers out while pointing the thumbs toward the toes. With the head up and while looking up, hold this position while inhaling and exhaling deeply. Hold the breath after each inhalation and exhalation, and with each exhalation relax deeper into the pose.

10.   Standing Forward Bend

This is a repeat of post No. 3. Come up to a standing position and bring both feet together. Place both hands at the sides of the feet while keeping the fingers extended forward and the thumbs extended back. Straighten the knees as much as possible while placing the nose between the knees. Exhale as deeply as possible and with each exhalation, go deeper into the pose by bending forward more and straightening the knees as much as possible.

11.   Upward Salute - Backward Bend

This is a repeat of pose No. 2. Bring both hands up above and bend backwards in the shape of the letter C. It took several years of daily practice before I was able to achieve good form with this pose, so be patient and do not force. While bending back as much as possible, inhale deeply and hold before exhaling.

12.   Mountain Pose

Stand up straight, inhale, exhale and enjoy the feeling of the body being awake and energized.

Step 5 - Corpse Pose

Lay on your back with the feet slightly apart, the arms at your side and the palms of the hands facing up. Begin slow and deep breathing, while systematically relaxing each part of the body beginning with the toes. Once the toes are relaxed, move on to the feet, and proceed to relax every part of the body. Try to keep the mind from racing and keep inner talking to a minimum. This a great pose to learn to clear and focus the mind, and to listen to the body. Remain in this pose for 10 – 15 minutes each day and the benefits will be noticed. With practice, the heart rate will be reduced along with the stress and tension of everyday life.

The Handstand

The handstand is an advanced exercise that requires a great deal of arm and upper body strength. This pose increases pressure on the blood vessels in the brain, therefore the handstand is not for everyone and it should be approached with extreme caution, if at all. My brother-in-law Dr. Bob Hammond (formerly with the NIH) has repeatedly warned against continuing to do the handstand as I age, but I find the benefits are too good to pass up. Fresh blood to the brain and the draining of blood from the legs every morning, seem to be vitally helpful in staving off the aging process. This is an upper body exercise that will help stave off the "shrinking chest syndrome" which is common as men age. Performing this pose after deep breathing will have an even greater benefit, as the increased flow of blood to the brain will be supercharged with oxygen.

I have been doing the handstand for many years, and even long before I was diagnosed with MS. Nolan Ryan's "Use It or Lose It" philosophy also proved an inspiration to never stop practicing the handstand. My 86-year-old Aunt Peggy, who recently retired from her incredible 50 hour-work-week job, has a pillow that says, "If I Rest, I'll Rust." Therefore, I have no plans to ever stop my handstands or exercise – at any point in my life.

I practice the handstand before weight training and chin-ups, because of any risk of muscle fatigue during the latter two. I do my daily handstand against the wall for a minimum of 30 seconds and for a maximum of 60 seconds. At the time of this writing, I am in the infancy of learning the coordination of balancing on my hands without wall support, and credit for the improvement of this skill goes to Christine Van Loo of the Cirque de la

Symphonie. When this company performs their unique blend of ballet and gymnastics with the Philadelphia Orchestra, it is a privilege to watch the unbelievable things these incredible athletes are able to do with their bodies. Christine has learned the rare ability to bridge the gap between the mind and the body which means that her gymnastic skills are limited only by her imagination.

Our two organizations performed together four years ago in Saratoga, NY. During a rehearsal break, I introduced myself and asked Christine if she would help me to balance on my hands. In addition to being a brilliant gymnast, Christine is also a talented and skilled teacher. When Christine performs a handstand, it appears effortless because she has discovered the easy way to do it. During our short lesson, she made it seem so easy, so I now devote daily time to the handstand, in search of that easy way to balance on my hands. Once a season I am fortunate to get a checkup with Christine to help with handstand form and keep me pointed in the right direction.

The process of learning to balance on my hands is a reminder of the time when I was learning to balance on a bicycle without training wheels. Before I understood how to balance on two wheels it seemed impossible, just as balancing on my hands seems now. I cannot reliably balance on my hands today, but that does not mean I will not reliably balance on my hands tomorrow. An autographed copy of Nando Parrado's book, *Miracle in the Andes*, is kept on display in my music studio, and his inscription reads: "Never, never give up."

MS Weight Training

My third MS attack in August 1999 stripped away most of my physical strength and endurance. Walking the distance of a single city block required all my energy, and it rendered me exhausted and out of breath. Even small physical activities sapped my strength, and they elevated my pulse to the point my entire central nervous system was affected. With an unwillingness to accept what was happening, I began mental preparations for the fight of my life. Following the heavy doses of steroids and the time it took for my central nervous system to calm down, my vision improved to a point where I was able to read. At that point, I was fortunate to have found two books that would be game changers in my recovery.

The first book was *Nolan Ryan's Pitcher's Bible*, which was originally purchased to help my son learn to pitch for his Little League team and the second book, *A Practical Approach to Strength Training*, by Matt Brzycki, was one that was stumbled upon while leisurely browsing in a bookstore. Both books are excellent and they were instrumental in helping to plan a strategy that would condition and strengthen my body without stressing or overheating my weak and fragile central nervous system. *Nolan Ryan's Pitcher's Bible* deals with weight training along with many other exercises, and *A Practical Approach to Strength Training* deals primarily with weight training. Both books focus on exercises for the body, but they also offer valuable information about psychology and an understanding of how the brain controls the body.

With the guidance of both books, I began experimenting with weights and came up with a hybrid approach to lifting – what I call "MS Weight Training." This approach differs from traditional weight training which is commonly based on repetitions to build muscle mass as well as strength. MS Weight Training is based on a simple notion of lifting, holding and breathing. The wrists, elbows and shoulders enjoy an advantage from this system because they are not subjected to repeated stressful movements under heavy loads of weight, which reduce the likelihood of strains and injuries. MS Weight Training, which is a hybrid approach that combines yoga and traditional weight lifting, also proved to be highly effective in building muscle strength without unwanted muscle mass.

One other benefit was a complete lack of sweat while weightlifting. I ruled out any workout that raised my body temperature to the point of sweating, so this approach effectively addressed that issue while rebuilding strength. My livelihood as a professional cellist could easily be adversely affected by unwanted muscle mass or injuries to the wrists, elbows and shoulders. Therefore the lift and hold approach was free of injuries and it built "smart muscles" instead of bulky ones. I always do my weightlifting immediately following my morning yoga session because that is when the muscles, joints, ligaments and tendons are warmed up and limber. My mind is sharper in the morning after deep breathing, so that is also the best time to avoid mishaps when working with weights.

Equipment Needed for Lifting Weights

1. An adjustable weight bench. When lifting weights, safety is top priority. Therefore choose a strong and stable weight bench that features widely placed feet and built in safety spotters. I do not recommend locating the weight bench in a damp musty basement because deep breathing is a major part of this system of working with weights. Deep breathing moldy air in a damp basement can create more problems than weight training will solve.

2. A set of adjustable dumbbells with weight up to 50 lbs. each.

3. A weight bar and a set of weights. I recommend building strength with 5 lb. plates, so weight can be added gradually.

4. A set of padded weightlifting gloves. Gnarled grips on a weight bar have a way of wreaking havoc with the palms of the hands, so the use of gloves will protect the palms and guard against heavy weights slipping out of sweaty hands. As a cellist, I would never consider working with weights without gloves.

I will admit to purchasing an Olympic set of weights and an Olympic weight bench after reading *Nolan Ryan's Pitcher's Bible*. This is the exact equipment Nolan used during his workouts, and my thinking was not to emulate Nolan Ryan, but to become Nolan Ryan. The concept may seem strange, but my goal was not to imitate the people who accomplished the impossible – it was to become those people. Becoming another person is not realistic, but I will admit Nolan Ryan is one person I would have been happy to become. Remember, the best actors are not the ones who simply act the role – the best actors are those who become the role. The same philosophy applies to fighting MS; therefore becoming someone who accomplished the impossible will be an advantageous mindset in the battle.

My initial MS Weight Training progressed at a very slow pace, with only dumbbells and free weights and with very light weight. Before MS, I had good upper body strength, but now it was a struggle to bench press only a 45 pound Olympic bar with no weights added. Those initial attempts at weightlifting gave little reason for optimism, but with time, the weights began to feel lighter and my confidence increased along with my strength. When I was able to lift the bar without difficulty, I added 5 lb. plates to both sides of the bar over the next few months. After approximately two years, I achieved my goal of benching the Olympic bar with a single 45 lb. plate on each end, for a total weight of 135 lbs. My objective during MS Weight Training was not to be an Olympic competitor or a body builder – it was only to rebuild my strength. This is another exercise that counters the "shrinking chest syndrome" which is often an accepted part of the aging process for men.

Step 1 - The Bench Press

Lie on the bench and grip the bar. This should not be attempted without a spotter or a weight bench with good built in spotters that will catch the bar. Dropping a heavy weighted bar on your chest or your neck could very well render MS a moot point. Grip the bar, inhale deeply, and slowly lift the bar while exhaling. Hold the bar with the arms extended, but not hyperextended, while breathing slowly and deeply. Then slowly lower the bar down onto the rack. Repeat this one or two times before moving on to sitting curls. Now that I am back at full strength, I lower the bar only halfway after benching, and I hold it at that height for as long as possible. Avoiding shaking muscles while holding a weighted Olympic bar will be difficult at first, but this will also get easier over time.

Step 2 - The Sitting Curl

Sit on the bench with the back straight and place one dumbbell in the right hand with the palm facing up, and resting down between the knees. With the weight in one hand, slowly curl the dumbbell up to the chest and hold while breathing deeply. Slowly lower the dumbbell down while continuing the deep breathing. Repeat this several times then switch hands to balance the workout. It is vital to continue the deep breathing as this will oxygenate the muscles and help to build tone and strength. I also recommend gradually increasing the weight as improving strength allows.

Step 3 - The Bent-Over Row

This exercise is a rowing motion but when lifting the dumbbell it should be rotated 180 degrees. Stand to the left side of the bench and place the right lower leg and knee and the right hand on the seat of the bench. With the left hand, reach down to the floor and grab hold of one dumbbell. Lift the dumbbell to chest level while twisting counterclockwise and hold for a count of 10 before slowly lowering. Be sure to breathe deeply while lifting, holding and lowering the dumbbell. Repeat this 2 – 3 times then switch to the opposite side of the bench while reversing the position lifting with the right hand - twisting clockwise with the right hand. Repeat this 2 – 3 times as well.

Step 4 - MS Chin-ups

Each morning I do chin-ups after my handstands and weight training. A handstand should not be attempted after weight lifting or chin-ups because muscle fatigue during a handstand could easily result in a surprise trip to the hospital, therefore the handstand should precede weight training or chin-ups. An accident during a handstand or the bench press could be problematic, but if your hands slip off the chin-up bar, there is a good chance of landing on your feet.

Chin-ups are part of my daily routine but my MS system comprises only one chin-up and one pull-up. These are done by going up very slowly over 10 seconds, and then holding for 10 seconds with my legs extended straight out in front. Then I come back down very slowly over 10 seconds. Even one slow-motion chin-up is a challenging workout. This method came from my one and only session with a personal trainer many years ago. During the session, she had me count to ten while doing a slow chin-up, then count to ten while coming down. The wisdom of that always stayed with me and I applied it to weightlifting after reading *Nolan Ryan's Pitcher's Bible.* In his book, Nolan refers to the benefits of developing balance skills while working with free weights. Performing extremely slow chin-ups also reduces any unnecessary wear and tear on the joints that would occur during repetitive motion under heavy weight. The objective is not to stress the joints, but to strengthen everything around them.

Stair Climbing

My regular commute to the orchestra involves the half-mile bike ride to the train station, day or night, followed by a short run up the 45 steps to the top of the elevated train platform. I run up the 45 steps two steps at a time for the purpose of maintaining stamina and coordination. The inspiration for running up steps on a regular basis is Nolan Ryan once again. Part of his regular workout involved running up the steps of the baseball stadium. If this part of his routine helped him stave off the aging process for 25 years, then it could certainly help with MS. Keep in mind, my run up the steps is only for a short distance, and that brief run does not give my body a chance to sweat or cause the cardiovascular system to run hot.

Chapter 32

Achieving the Placebo Effect – Step-by-Step

This book would not be complete without detailing exactly how I was able to learn the power of the placebo effect. Excellent books have been written by those who specialize in treating MS and by those who have successfully accepted the disease as a life-long partner. There are also good books written by those who have managed to get the disease into remission and books by others who have lost the battle. Yet, I have never read a book by someone who has beaten the disease and provided a detailed systematic process of exactly how it was accomplished.

Meditation

Daily meditation is vital but it will only be effective if practiced together with a proper diet and a trim and physically fit body. The true purpose of a disciplined diet and exercise regimen is to prepare the body for the role of the soldier who follows orders from Central Command. Without Central Command, a soldier lacks guidance and discipline, just as our bodies lack guidance and discipline without orders from the brain. MS and many other diseases attack the body, however the battle against many of these diseases will be fought in the mind. Therefore understanding and accepting this is the key to unlocking the mystery behind the placebo effect. Without a proper diet and exercise, it will not be possible for the body to be under complete control of the mind, and victory will remain elusive. Meditation will succeed only when the body is ready for the mind to take command.

Repeating a series of commands on a regular basis over a long period is an effective way to train the brain to make physical changes in the body. To quell any doubts about the brain's ability to make such changes, one needs only to look at the unexplained success in the clinical trial placebo groups. Cells of the human body are constantly dying and being replaced, so why can't the brain have some say in the makeup of those replacement cells? Around the time of my third attack, I was given the book, *You the Healer*, by Jose Silva and Robert B. Stone. The book is excellent as it details ways of training the mind to make changes to the body. I firmly believe this is the ability that is unknowingly possessed by people who achieve the placebo effect. After studying what the Silva Method has to offer, I came up with a system that enabled me to acquire the desired degree of mental control.

The human brain is essentially a computer that processes information, but what makes the brain stand out is its ability to think and reason on its own. For any computer to function, it is necessary to have a program or a set of instructions to follow, and in this sense, the human brain is similar. If the brain is successfully programmed to achieve specific tasks with the body, the possibilities become endless. We all have the ability to program the brain to some degree, and programming the brain is a skill that can be honed and improved just like any other skill. Brainwashing is a good example. Isn't brainwashing a methodical way of programming someone else's brain to follow a given set of instructions? Consider physical coordination, which is mind over muscle. An athlete will drill a play to be used in sports competition, or an instrumentalist will drill a difficult passage to be performed in concert. These are examples of training the muscles, but to a greater degree they are learned motor memory skills. Learning such skills may seem like an intensive physical process, but it is actually programming of the human brain.

The following is a list of the commands that I repeated for two 30-minute sessions every day for a period of more than two years, and I began this practice shortly after my vicious and debilitating third MS attack. Mental commands should be practiced in a quiet environment that is free of distractions. In addition to repeating commands silently, it is important to visualize the process of each command as it takes place. Detailed, vivid images and mental videos of each event should be displayed and viewed in the mind.

The Repeated Meditation Commands

1. I see and feel the MS going into remission and leaving my body.

While repeating this command, I envisioned a scene from a Civil War battlefield. During intense fighting, MS was taking heavy flanking fire and suffering large numbers of casualties. MS underestimated me as an opponent and it retreated while waving the white flag.

2. I see and feel all lesions in my brain and spinal cord disappearing and all damaged tissue regenerating.

The multitude of lesions in my brain and the huge one in my spinal cord were causing so much trouble, so I devised this command to address and resolve the issue. During the first part of this command, I watched each lesion evaporating into a mist, and for the second part, I watched the healing process take place in the brain and spinal cord. Years later when I saw my MRIs from 2013, they were eerily similar to what I envisioned while repeating this one command.

3. I see and feel the optic nerves regenerating and my eyesight returning.

I gave special attention to my optic nerves because the loss of my eyesight was an even greater concern than losing the use of my hands. Without my hands, playing the cello was the main problem but losing my eyesight posed a serious threat to a normal everyday life. During meditation I visualized both inflamed optic nerves calming down and returning to normal. I also envisioned them regenerating to normalcy where they were sending full transmissions from the eyes to the brain. It is interesting to note my right optic nerve fully recovered, but my left one returned only to where it was before the third attack.

4. I see and feel the use of my hands and fingers returning with new and improved coordination skills.

I was determined to regain the complete use of my hands because the ability to play the cello was not going to be taken away. In addition to meditating this command, I devoted a great deal of time and energy to my many forms of physical therapy for both the hands and fingers. It is my belief that we should never wait for the body to heal; we have to make it heal.

5. I see and feel the brain finding new and improved pathways to the muscles.

While meditating instructions for the brain to find new pathways to the muscles, I visualized a color roadmap that displayed new routes from the brain to the muscles. The resulting images resembled a simulated route on a GPS on the slowest setting. This was before the time of the GPS, but I actually watched the slow progress of the brain navigating the trip.

I repeated each command several times, but with a pause between each repeat where I continued to visualize each command coming to fruition. If one has the discipline (or the desperation) to practice this for two 30-minute sessions every day for two years, there is no limit to what can be accomplished. A positive mental attitude is a must. Practicing these meditative commands as a non-believer will result in 60 minutes of wasted time each day.

The above list was for my specific needs but the repeated commands should be customized to each individual's case. MS will affect the muscle control and the central nervous system differently with each person, so the repeated commands should be customized to address how and where MS has affected each individual.

Keep in mind that repeated meditative commands will only be effective if they are practiced in conjunction with diet, exercise, stress reduction and discipline. The culmination of all these factors will enable the brain to learn the ability to make changes in the body. In the West, we know yoga largely as a form of physical exercise, but it goes much deeper. Yoga is an ancient art form that raises the mind and consciousness to a spiritual level, and the poses and lifestyle serve to condition the body to enable the freeing of the mind. Advanced yogis are masters of what I have only begun to accomplish. I have devoted only a few years to meditation and a disciplined lifestyle, but true yogis devote a lifetime to the practice.

Chapter 33

Make it Official

My Last Visit with Dr. Markowitz Prior to the Eleven-Year Sabbatical

My appointment with Dr. Markowitz on November 20, 2002, was the last time I would see him until May 2013, almost eleven years later. Some reasons for the long hiatus were based on fear and others were because of my extreme stubbornness. At that last visit in 2002, Dr. Markowitz administered some basic neurological tests and the results were quite good, then he told me to walk across the room and back. Remembering how unsteady my walking skills were just three years earlier, he remarked that I was much better. I replied, "Much better? Watch this…" In the center of the room, I squatted and placed both hands flat on the floor, then slowly pushed myself up into an unassisted handstand. I thought Dr. Markowitz might be impressed, but his reaction was unexpected. He said, "Wait here," and left the room for several minutes and returned with five people I assumed were neurologists or residents. Then Dr. Markowitz looked at me and said, "Do that again." After successfully performing the circus trick for his audience, they congratulated me and left the room.

Dr. Markowitz then sat down with pen and pad in hand, and asked exactly what I was doing with diet, exercise and supplements. As I told of my research, the discoveries and my disciplined lifestyle, Dr. Markowitz sat writing feverishly. He then said an entire set of new MRIs of my brain and spinal cord would be needed to see what was going on. I nodded my head in agreement, but there was no way I was going to subject my body to more MRIs or any other tests.

Before leaving, I broached the subject of the placebo effect. I asked Dr. Markowitz for his opinion on the unusually high success rates in the clinical trial placebo groups of MS drugs. Dr. Markowitz believes that behind the placebo effect is some chemical produced by the brain that causes changes in the body. I asked, "What is that chemical?" and he replied, "I don't know, but I wish I could bottle it and give it to all my patients." I said, "I'm going to find out what that chemical is."

I did not see Dr. Markowitz again for the next eleven years, and much of that time was spent searching for that elusive chemical. A curious thing about that November 2002 visit was the very last thing Dr. Markowitz said to me. As he entered his final notes in my chart, Dr. Markowitz looked up and said with a smile, "Okay, you're cured."

When I met Nando Parrado on April 15, 2013, I sensed a strange and intense energy radiating from this powerful man. He had accomplished the impossible. At that moment I had a distinct feeling my MS had not just gone into remission – it felt like I had totally cured myself of the disease. Had I actually gained membership in the club of those who had done the impossible? It had been thirteen and a half years since my last attack. During that time, I was completely asymptomatic. Meeting Nando provided the impetus and the inspiration to prove I was really cured, and to complete an unfinished book.

To officially call it a cure, it would be necessary to get tangible proof that others could see for themselves. After several weeks of hesitation, I called Dr. Markowitz to set up an appointment or a meeting of some kind. Much had changed for Dr. Markowitz during that eleven-year period. He had risen to prominence in the world of neurology, and he was no longer accepting new patients. I left a message with his receptionist about the news of my recovery, and it apparently piqued his interest. That day I received a return call from the receptionist, saying Dr. Markowitz very much wanted to see me. It would be our first meeting in eleven years.

In 1999, I had seen my family doctor, an orthopedic surgeon, a neurosurgeon, a neuro-ophthalmologist and five neurologists, and my last appointment with Dr. Markowitz was November 20, 2002. Dr. Markowitz is a superb neurologist, but after that visit, I needed a complete break from all neurologists, doctors, hospitals, MRIs, blood work and medications. My only contact with Dr. Markowitz's office during my 11 year sabbatical was when I called his receptionist for renewal scripts for Avonex®. In September 2003, I stopped taking the Avonex® and for the next ten years, there was no contact with Dr. Markowitz, his office or any other neurologist.

Hello Again, Dr. Markowitz!

The first time I saw Dr. Markowitz in August 1999, I was too sick and debilitated to be angry. In many ways, my body was reduced to a useless shell, and I was unable to do things that I had always taken for granted. I sat in his office, partially blind, unable to use my hands and barely able to walk. I was also partially incontinent and suffering from MS-related motion sickness. Up to that time, I had been clinging to a forlorn hope that MS was a misdiagnosis, but that hope evaporated with the unveiling of the numerous brain and spinal cord lesions in my 1999 MRI's.

My waist felt like it was fitted with a tight girdle and my entire body felt like it was receiving non-stop electric current. The "girdle effect" or the "MS Hug" made my life very uncomfortable. The condition is caused by an involuntary contraction of the muscles between the ribs. My abdomen constantly felt like I was wearing a girdle that had been pulled too tightly. The sensation of electric current in my neck, torso and arms is known as Lhermitte's Sign, which is named after the French neurologist Jean Lhermitte, who first documented the condition in 1924.

When I bent my head down, there was an intense sensation of electric current running down my spine. I also felt the same sensation on my shoulders and back after taking a hot shower. Lhermitte's Sign happens when scarring is formed in place of damaged or destroyed myelin. The nerves are then unable to properly send and receive signals from the brain. This condition is not limited to MS. It can also occur from spinal cord injuries, inflammation in the spinal cord, and even a severe deficiency of Vitamin B12.

To add insult to injury, I was hearing the constant sound of helicopters. MS can affect every part of the central nervous system in bizarre ways including the sense of hearing, and the unwanted sound of helicopter blades chopping the air is one of them. The first time I mentioned this to a doctor, who shall remain anonymous in this case, I was told to "go see a psychiatrist."

MS symptoms that affect hearing are uncommon. Sound is transmitted by the nerves along the auditory pathways to the brain. Therefore the sense of hearing is not spared from attacks by the disease. It is important to remember that MS does not affect any two people the same way. In rare cases where MS does affect the hearing, it is usually in the form of actual hearing loss. There are people with MS who have been known to experience my identical symptoms of hearing helicopter blades constantly chopping the air.

Bladder and bowel problems will affect at least 80% of people with MS. When there is an incontinence issue urinating, it is known as a neurogenic bladder. This condition happens when control of the bladder is compromised due to nerve damage. When the nerves are not able to respond to the commands of the brain, the muscles cannot respond. MS is a common culprit behind a neurogenic bladder, but the condition can also be caused by an injury or even a brain issue. Bowel problems can be serious or just sensory as they were in my case. Living on a natural diet was particularly helpful when dealing with this condition. With proper treatment and care, both issues are generally manageable.

Sitting in the waiting area of the HUP Department of Neurology for the first time in eleven years brought back those painful memories from the most difficult year of my life, but several things had radically changed since that time. The big difference was that the tables had turned. I was now the plaintiff and MS had become the defendant. After several minutes of reflecting on the past, a nurse called my name and took me to a health check station where she asked a series of questions and checked my vitals. Next, I was seen by Dr. Salim Chahin, a neurologist who works with Dr. Markowitz. Dr. Chahin had some prior knowledge of my case, as he was familiar with my records and MRIs from 1999. He gave me a neurological examination that included everything from touching the tip of my nose with one finger to telling him when the base of a tuning fork stopped vibrating on my hand while my eyes were closed. Dr. Chahin seemed surprised at how well the tests went, but he seemed puzzled that a person debilitated by a severe case of MS and with so many lesions could make a complete recovery.

He asked what I had done – then probably regretted asking, because I spoke at infomercial speed for the next five minutes in an attempt to condense eleven years of history into several minutes. Dr. Chahin then expressed an interest in seeing current MRIs of my brain and spinal cord, but I explained that I had already decided to decline the tests. Without any debate, he smiled and said he would return with Dr. Markowitz. I was somewhat apprehensive of how Dr. Markowitz would greet me after the eleven-year hiatus, but when he entered the room with that same baby face, we shook hands and he seemed genuinely happy to see me again. I was ready to burst with childhood excitement, as I could not wait to tell him about the book I was writing and everything I had accomplished during the last eleven years.

After Dr. Markowitz inquired about the happenings of more than a decade, he listened to a condensed synopsis of the steps I had taken which resulted in my complete recovery. I told him about the writing of my book which had shifted into overdrive since meeting Nando Parrado. It came as no surprise when Dr. Markowitz explained the need to see new MRIs of my brain and spinal cord. He spoke of the advances in MRI technology over the past fourteen years and said how important it was to get updated MRIs with the contrast agent gadolinium. Because my system had been subjected to so many tests and drugs fourteen years earlier, I explained there would be no more MRIs and no contrast agent injected into my veins. During that 1999 year from hell I endured six MRIs, a bone scan, x-rays, a nerve conduction velocity test, a horribly unpleasant spinal tap, three tests for lime disease, heavy metal toxicity tests, a multitude of visual field tests, and countless blood tests.

My MS may have been a textbook case in many ways, but it was unprecedented for a person with such a severe case to make a complete recovery. Before this visit it was a given that Dr. Markowitz would insist on a new series of MRIs complete with gadolinium, but I had already made up my mind to forego the procedure. The official reason for declining the MRIs was to not subject my body to more of the tests and injections that had been endured fourteen years earlier, but the real reason for declining the MRIs was out of fear of any hidden secrets that might be revealed. I had been completely asymptomatic for fourteen years and was living a completely normal life, and in many ways, it was the life of an amateur athlete. After listening to my reasons Dr. Markowitz refused to take no for an answer, and he gave two convincing reasons for having the MRIs:

1. As my neurologist, he needed to see exactly what was going on in my brain and spinal cord.

2. It would be unethical to write a book about beating MS without seeing the MRIs that showed proof of what I had accomplished.

I told him I would discuss this with my wife, but from that moment, it was clear there was no choice in the matter. I had prepared a lengthy argument to firmly stand my ground and decline the MRIs, but Dr. Markowitz's logical reasoning overruled anything that I had previously decided. The next day I called the HUP Department of Radiology and scheduled the MRIs.

Chapter 34

The MRI Machine Awaits

Returning to the HUP Department of Radiology after fourteen years brought back even more unsettling memories. Many unpleasant experiences from 1999 had been deleted from memory for reasons of self-preservation, but some of those memories slowly began to reemerge. Revisiting those dormant scenes from 1999 was initially painful, but the unpleasantness was short-lived. A sudden realization emerged that the purpose of my presence at HUP was to prove I had cured myself of MS. The understanding of that notion gave me a feeling of control, and I began to believe the results of my MRIs would be positive.

In preparation for an MRI at HUP, all patients are taken to a room, assigned a locker to store their belongings and issued a tired-looking hospital gown. There are separate rooms for men and women, so I was placed in a room with seven other men. Several of them seemed to be dealing with very serious health issues. After seeing other patients in a bad way, I felt truly fortunate to have reclaimed my life by turning the tables on MS. My mind was racing with anxiety about my first MRI in fourteen years, so after changing into my gown I took a seat with my laptop and tried to clear my head with some writing.

After a two-hour wait, my name was called and I was escorted to the MRI room where an attractive young red haired radiologist began an interrogation with a series of questions that included everything from health and medication history to issues of claustrophobia. She offered an MP3 player along with a set of headphones, but I declined and told her of my skill to withdraw into my own world, away from any situation. Once on the MRI table, I did accept a set of earplugs to protect against the prolonged and intense high volume of an MRI machine. A technician then instructed me to lie motionless for the next hour then slid my entire body into the machine. It is understandable how people can feel claustrophobic while being confined to a deafening narrow tube for one hour, but when the noise started, I began meditating positive thoughts and entered a state-of-mind where I left my physical body. At some point, my dream state changed to one of deep sleep, and I was rudely awakened by a male MRI technician who apparently felt it necessary to check in and see how I was doing. I was annoyed at him for unnecessarily disrupting my slumber, but with a degree of self-control, I politely said I would notify him if I needed anything. Perhaps someone should have had the foresight to equip MRI machines with a "Do Not Disturb" sign.

The next interruption was for part two of the MRI. I was injected with the contrast agent gadolinium. They slid me out of the MRI tube only halfway so it was impossible to lift my head to see what was going on. A mystery medical resident whom I never saw then skillfully injected the gadolinium into my arm with no mishap. Suddenly I remembered an episode from one of my six MRIs in 1999, when a medical resident who was apparently exhausted from an overnight shift, administered my gadolinium injection. This tired young man inserted the needle into my arm but missed the vein and injected the gadolinium into the muscle in my forearm. For the following week, I had a painfully bruised arm and little to smile about. After the latest successful gadolinium injection, I was placed back into the MRI tube for part two. The deafening sounds of the MRI resumed where they left off, and once again, I quickly withdrew into a deep meditative state.

My next awakening came when I was slid out of the tube at the conclusion of the MRI, and I was somehow sad to see that relaxing hour come to an end. In a great mood and feeling victorious, I returned to the men's waiting room to retrieve my clothes and belongings from the locker. There would be no celebrating just yet because there was a long two-month wait before I would see the results of these MRIs at the next follow up visit with Dr. Markowitz.

Chapter 35

"You did the impossible."

"The person who says something is impossible should not interrupt the person doing it."

- Chinese Proverb

During the drive to HUP for the follow-up of my June 2013 MRI, I was accompanied by some unwanted anxiety. I felt great physically but I was fearful of what secrets might be divulged by the spinal cord and brain. During the past fourteen years I may have been totally asymptomatic, but there was no way of knowing what surprises would show up on the latest MRIs. After arriving at the neurology wing and signing in, I took a seat in the waiting area and began deep breathing in an attempt to calm my racing mind. When my name was called a nurse escorted me to her health check station where I was once again asked a series of rather personal questions. Then she checked my weight, pulse and blood pressure. When she asked what medications I was taking I felt so proud to brag that I was on no medications, but she did not seem the least bit interested. With a poker face, she dryly gave instructions to have a seat and wait for Dr. Markowitz.

After a short wait, Dr. Chahin appeared and took me to an examination room. After several minutes of reviewing my chart, he conducted the standard neurological tests and instructed me to walk down the hallway and back. He said everything looked fine, but for some reason I felt compelled to show off for him with a handstand. After removing my shoes, I went up into a handstand against the wall and took both feet off the wall while balancing on my hands for about 15 seconds. Dr. Chahin looked totally puzzled and said, "That's amazing!" He then wanted to know how I was able to do a handstand. I explained the handstand is part of my daily four S's: S***, shower, shave and stretch!

When Dr. Markowitz entered the room, I repeated the handstand demonstration and he said, "I wish I could do that." Dr. Markowitz sat down and brought up the most recent MRIs on his computer screen and after looking them over he said, "You made a 99 percent improvement." It took a moment to sink in, and then he looked at me with a serious face and said, "You did the impossible." The anxiety I felt on the way to the appointment was replaced with a sudden euphoria. I had climbed thirty-seven and a half miles through the Andes Mountains with no equipment, supplies or training. I just blew a fastball by the batter for strike three and the final out of my seventh no hitter. The World Chess Championship title had been wrested from the Soviets and it was in my hands. I felt like my son Ryan, the MMA fighter, when he rendered his opponent Ryan Holmes (the nephew of World Boxing Champion Larry Holmes) unconscious with a guillotine choke hold 26 seconds into the first round.

I did not win any principal cello auditions during my recovery but having Dr. Markowitz award me the gold medal of neurological achievements was even better. It was reminiscent of the moment on May 6, 1985, at the Philadelphia Orchestra's cello audition. The audition was over and nine of us who played in the final round were in the Green Room of the Academy of Music waiting for the results to be announced. The legendary principal French horn of the orchestra, Mason Jones, who was personnel manager of the orchestra at the time, entered the room to announce the audition results and the room fell silent. With his famous dry demeanor he announced, "The Committee chose Cafaro."

The current announcement by Dr. Markowitz was great, but even better was the fact that a highly respected neurologist in the medical world had now given credence to what I had devoted my heart and soul, and the last fourteen years of my life, to accomplishing. Dr. Markowitz brought up the subject of my MRIs from 1999, and with his uncanny memory he said, "Your scan fourteen years ago was really ugly. I remember it was quite impressive as everything in your brain was lighting up." He was not exaggerating because I later counted 53 lesions in the brain, and the huge angry 3.5 cm lesion in my neck. I walked out of the office smiling because the MS had left with its tail between its legs.

Meeting Nando Parrado was truly inspirational for moving ahead with this book, but hearing such a highly respected neurologist at the Hospital of the University of Pennsylvania say I did the impossible was equally powerful. I had run the proverbial sub-four-minute MS mile, and I had been given a green light to show others how I did it. I have no doubt my record will be short lived, and I hope to watch others shave the seconds off my record. Beating MS was considered impossible, but now that I had actually accomplished it, it was high time to get serious by finishing the book and helping others to break my record.

November 22, 2013 - My First Visit with Dr. Sergott in Fourteen Years

A period of eleven years elapsed where I did not see Dr. Markowitz, but it was fourteen years since I saw Dr. Sergott. Much had changed at Wills Eye Hospital since 1999. Dr. Sergott had been elevated from a top neuro-ophthalmologist at Wills Eye Hospital in Philadelphia, to the head of the Department of Neuro-Ophthalmology. I was in such a state of denial for so many years that I avoided going back to any of the doctors I had seen in 1999. Drs. Sperling, Lublin, DeHoratius, Sergott, and Markowitz are all excellent, but I was unable to deal with the truth and I wanted different answers. For my fourteen-year reunion with Dr. Sergott, I came equipped with a CD of my complete MRIs from five months earlier that showed no lesions in the brain or spinal cord, and no signs of MS.

As the head of the Department of Neuro-Ophthalmology at Wills Eye Hospital and a renowned MS specialist, Dr. Sergott is understandably busy and in very high demand. It took two months to get an appointment, but it was well worth the wait. This meeting was an emotional moment in my life because Dr. Sergott gave a warm hug and a smile, and said how happy he was to see me doing so well after all those years. The euphoria of seeing him fascinated with my beating of MS took me back to my childhood when I proudly showed off my newly learned skill of riding a bicycle without training wheels. I sat at Dr. Sergott's desk as he viewed my MRIs on his computer screen, and I watched his facial expressions as he compared the images from 1999 and 2013. This was even better than balancing on two wheels; it felt like I was showing off advanced cycling skills of extended wheelies and bunny hopping. His face took on a look of seriousness when he asked exactly what I did during those years to have completely beaten such a severe case of MS.

After he listened to my lengthy summary, we discussed my book and he advised against giving credit to any one particular thing, because he believes the culmination of everything I did was responsible for the success. It was great to see him again after all these years because I was now seeing him on my terms. I thanked him for his words fourteen years earlier when he said those memorable words that changed my outlook and future. Having the chance to thank him personally for giving me hope at my darkest hour was great, but seeing the bright smile it brought to his face was even better. I reiterated his words of seeing patients in a hopeless condition one year later who were still in a wheelchair, and other patients one year later and he didn't know anything was wrong with them. Dr. Sergott beamed when I told him I had looked up "bedside manners" in the dictionary and saw his picture. We talked about the brain lesions on the MRIs and that mean looking lesion in my spinal cord. He was very impressed with what I had accomplished. Dr. Sergott then displayed his exemplary skills as a doctor and human being when he asked how he could get that same help for others who are in need.

The most precious moment in our meeting was when I expressed to Dr. Sergott how grateful I was for his words of hope fourteen years ago. His humble response was, "Are you kidding? You not only made my day, you just made my decade!" A doctor with his level of passion is not one who merely goes to work for a paycheck. Dr. Sergott is a person who is intensely devoted to helping people under his care, and he will never stop searching for answers.

Meeting Jodi Gelfand for the First Time in Fourteen Years

"During the first year with an illness, the real battle is not with your disease but with your brain."

- Jodi Gelfand

It had been fourteen years since I saw Jodi. On an evening of a Philadelphia Orchestra concert at Carnegie Hall, we sat across from each other over dinner in a healthy restaurant in New York City. Watching Jodi read excerpts in my book about our meeting fourteen earlier was yet one more of those magical moments. As she read excerpts from the book, I watched her expressions change from looks of astonishment to ear-to-ear smiles. It was a meeting I wished would never end, but nothing lasts forever.

"You did the impossible."

It only took a few days to get in touch with Jodi and she was more than happy to get together after fourteen years. It had been so long since we saw each other and I sat across the table the same distance as I sat across her desk in 1999. As we talked, I felt that familiar positive energy she had radiated in 1999. I remembered Jodi mainly from her helpful words long ago, but this meeting gave an understanding of who Jodi is and exactly how she was so helpful at a time I was in such desperate need. When we first met I only knew Jodi as a physician's assistant, but her powerful prophecy changed my mindset and my life. Did she honestly believe what she had told me fourteen years ago about following the five steps and never hearing from MS again in my lifetime? Something inside me needed to know for sure. Prior to specializing in holistic medicine, Jodi's former career was on the Wall Street treadmill, but the time arrived to evolve and make a career change to one that was in her blood. We discussed her powerful words from fourteen years earlier and Jodi spoke of how receptive I was when she threw me the lifeline.

Listening to her philosophy of living life at a higher level was fascinating. It offered an in-depth understanding of her reasoning and beliefs behind what she said to me at the lowest point of my life. As a person who is never done learning, Jodi inquired as to the details of exactly what I had done over the years to have completely beaten MS. As I described each step in detail, Jodi listened while fastidiously taking notes. The scenario was ironic because I had waited so long to sit down together and express my gratitude for what she had done for me. Here Jodi was busy learning from what I had accomplished.

The people in this book who were my guides are individuals who never gave up, and they will never give up learning or trying to improve themselves. When we hugged goodbye it was one of those moments I wanted to last forever. Jodi Gelfand is a truly evolved soul, and I now know her advice and prediction in 1999 was honest and from the heart.

Dr. Joan Oshinsky - 2013

Dr. Oshinsky's wizardry always remained in the back of my mind, and fourteen years later I managed to track her down. We spoke on the phone several times and the best part was listening to her reaction as she viewed my MRIs from 1999 and 2013 on my website. Dr. Oshinsky gasped as she scrolled through the ugly lesions on the 1999 MRIs, then she was in awe while viewing the 2013 images. When a doctor whom you truly respect looks at what you have done and says, "That's amazing," it has a way of putting one in a good mood for the next few days. I contacted Dr. Oshinsky several months later when I was in her area and tried to set up a meeting, but her busy schedule kept it from happening. Meeting up with the people who were instrumental in my complete recovery has become a passion of mine, and I hope to one day sit face-to-face with Dr. Oshinsky and discuss her brilliantly accurate call in 1999. I will always be a big fan of her neurological talents.

Winning the Lottery

My Uncle Dave is a wise and philosophical man, and he once taught me a valuable lesson when he explained that when a person is eating three meals a day and has a roof over their head, everything beyond that is merely numbers on a balance sheet. About one year ago, my wife Teresa and I were having one of our deep, soul-searching discussions, when she unexpectedly asked how my life would change if I won the lottery or came into unlimited wealth. After a moment of lengthy reflection, I realized nothing about my life would change. I was already living a dream life with the person I wanted to share it with. The simple diet I have adopted is more of a religion than a discipline, and over time, my taste buds have completely acclimated to the taste of pure food. Therefore, there would be no dietary changes. When I do eat in restaurants, the taste of food with high amounts of salt, fat or sugar is an unfamiliar and unpleasant experience.

Our home is located exactly one-half mile from the PATCO train that runs from South Jersey to Philadelphia, and the final stop on the line is one block from the Kimmel Center, which is the orchestra's home. Since our home is in such close proximity to the train, self-imposed house rules forbid driving the car to the station in all weather conditions, day or night. The bike trip from the house consumes exactly two minutes, and taking the car to the station actually adds time to the commute. Finding a parking space at the train station and walking from the car to the train platform increases the commuting time by at least ten minutes. Since I only bike to the station, there is little use for my car and there is no need or any desire for a new one. A new car would just grow old and lonely while sitting alone on the driveway.

Many people are lucky to have studied a musical instrument as a child, but I am one of the few who did not quit (thanks to Mom) and one of the rare ones who went on to a conservatory. If that is not enough, I am one of the chosen few lucky enough to play music for a living. Not only do I get to play

"You did the impossible."

the cello professionally, but also I have a position with the Philadelphia Orchestra, which is a legend in the world of music.

In life, there are two things: what you love to do and what you do for a living. If they are the same thing, it means God is smiling at you. I have the distinct feeling someone up there is smiling at me because I not only play the cello for a living, but I have been given my life back. When eyesight, use of the hands, the ability to walk and everything that is taken for granted is stripped away and then returned, it changes one's perception of life. Wealth would not change my life in any way because I no longer take anything for granted. This is my second chance at life and I have nothing to complain about and everything to be grateful for.

Chapter 36

Did I Really Cure Myself of MS?

I have spoken with several doctors who believe I must have been misdiagnosed with MS. Curing MS is not possible therefore they surmise I must have had something else. During my last visit with Dr. Markowitz this possibility was discussed and he said, "Because I did not follow your progress for eleven years, I cannot say for sure what you had." But when I left his office he handed me the paper to give to his receptionist, and on the line next to Diagnosis, he had written Multiple Sclerosis. Several of my colleagues in the Philadelphia Orchestra suggested I must have somehow ingested a poison, and this possibility was discussed with several doctors. The doctors I spoke with agree that poison could cause one or two of the symptoms I suffered, but it is not possible for any poison to have caused all of my symptoms.

Learning from a Great Teacher – MS

The battle against MS was the greatest and the most difficult learning experience of my life – it changed everything about me as a person. Despite all the hardships and suffering this disease brought into my life, I would not trade what I went through for anything in the world. The challenge of fighting this horrible illness taught me to look deep inside for answers and to use every past experience in life as a mentor and a guide. It is impossible to know what we are capable of unless we are called upon to face challenges that are beyond our abilities. It often takes an unfortunate and adversarial experience to learn just what we are capable of.

Had Nando Parrado missed his ill-fated flight to Chile, he may have turned out to be just another ordinary person from Uruguay who would never see snow. Jascha Heifetz received a negative review of a performance early in his career and it devastated him. The critic wrote how Heifetz's high standards were slipping and that he was letting down the public, letting himself down and letting down music itself. After that review, Heifetz committed to seriously devoting his life to music and to the unprecedented level of excellence that became his trademark. Had he not received such a critical review it is likely he would never have maintained his obsession with perfection that raised the standard of violin playing to an impossible level.

I was always fascinated by people who accomplished things considered to be impossible, but I never thought of myself as one of them. I now know how to handle a life-threatening illness, but I always wondered how I would fare in a life-threatening survival situation. Since my outdoor adventures are limited to cycling and hiking on marked trails, the chances are good I will never be put to the test. Being in a wilderness survival situation was admittedly one of my closet fantasies, but I can say with certainty that being in a survival situation against a major illness was not. As it turned out, the luck of the draw presented me with the test of surviving a brutal health crisis instead of a life-threatening situation in the wilderness.

The struggle against MS was the biggest obstacle I ever faced, and the lack of an established guidebook and the uncertainty of an outcome only served to compound what seemed like an impossible and never-ending task. It was delusional to think I would never deal with a health crisis before the ripe old age of 100, but the reality of being human struck hard and fast with my diagnosis. That rude awakening brought an understanding that each of us will more than likely deal with a major health crisis at some point, just as our homes and cars will eventually need major repairs. A proper diet, exercise and a disciplined lifestyle will do a great deal to stave off the aging process and maintain a good quality of life, but at some point the human body will begin to wear out and fail. I would love to say I will defeat any and all future health challenges, but that is not a possibility. At some point my mortal limits will greet me and then it will be time to meet my maker. At that point perhaps I can look forward to an eternity in the afterlife – with no health crises.

I've Cured Myself of MS – Now What?

Since seeing my 2013 MRIs that are totally clear of lesions, I admit to a growing temptation of being drawn back into the soft life. The desperate motivation to fight MS is gone and I no longer feel the omnipresent threat of that dreaded fourth attack eagerly waiting in the wings. With the euphoria of curing myself of MS, I have become slightly less disciplined about how much water I drink, and I have grown increasingly complacent about limiting the amount of food I eat. Since that time when Dr. Markowitz said I had done the impossible, my waistline has grown from an ideal 32 inches to 34 inches, and the pants I purchased to accommodate the extra width seem to be growing tighter.

The soft life is one of the biggest threats to our health and we all face it each day. Remember the first Energy Secretary of the United States, James Schlesinger, who said, "Americans have two modes – complacency and panic." Although I no longer live with MS, I somehow miss the constant challenge of the everyday fight. During my war with the disease, discipline at the dinner table was never an issue and it was easy to decline that second serving to ensure the sensation of hunger was present at bedtime. Now that my back is no longer against the wall, there is a new adversary I am dealing with, and it is the soft life. In some ways I understand what early retirement feels like and it is not something I am handling well. My Aunt Peggy's motto -"If I rest I'll rust"- seems to have taken on a new meaning. It has become clear I need a new challenge and a desire to stay hungry. All the people I credit with accomplishing the impossible had a talent for staying hungry and not growing complacent. The soft life has come softly knocking and it has managed to get one foot in the door. It may be hard to believe, but in some ways this latest challenge is proving to be a more difficult opponent than MS. During Nando Parrado's lecture in Philadelphia on April 15, 2013, he joked about how he was "a bit heavier" than he used to be. This was a clear example of a remarkable person who thrived in a life-threatening survival situation. He is no longer fighting for his life, therefore he has grown accustomed to many of life's luxuries.

The need for a challenge is something of a basic necessity, and only when we are faced with great challenges, will we know our capabilities and limits. Nando Parrado's challenge was facing certain death and with that challenge he showed no limits and displayed capabilities he probably never realized he possessed. When Heifetz received that bad review by a critic, he saw those words as the death of his artistry and from that point he devoted his life to fighting the musical Grim Reaper. A great interview with Jascha Heifetz is included with his extensive discography *The Heifetz Collection*. This fascinating interview offers an opportunity to listen to this great artist's views on the subject of discipline. Heifetz was a master of discipline and he is forthcoming about a lack of discipline in many of today's aspiring violinists. The great violinist and pedagogue Carl Flesch said Heifetz's intense level of discipline is what enabled him to successfully make that difficult transition from child prodigy to the adult master. Jascha Heifetz even said we almost have to refuse ourselves a few things in life because "We have too many comforts." James Ehnes is one of the truly great violinists of our time and he performs at a level of flawlessness that few instrumentalists could ever dream of achieving. He regularly appears as guest soloist with the Philadelphia Orchestra, and I always take advantage of the opportunity to speak with him backstage. At our most recent meeting I shared my cello teacher's firsthand story of how Jascha Heifetz warmed up by methodically drilling each passage in the concerto for two solid hours prior to the performance. The purpose of sharing this story was to confirm my assumption that Mr. Ehnes' standard of excellence was based on a similar practice regimen. It was a total surprise when he said, "Wow. I don't have that kind of discipline."

Nolan Ryan faced the challenge of the limits of the human body and the aging process, but he refused to accept those limits. Everything about his life including diet, exercise regimen and lifestyle, would be focused on expanding the limits of his body. When Bobby Fisher lost his first game to the Grandmaster Max Pavey at age nine, he cried like a baby, then decided he would do whatever it would take to become the world chess champion. Lance Armstrong faced an insurmountable health challenge and he was victorious. Although he is known today as a cheat and liar, it is important to focus on how he fought and beat his illness. How many people could be capable of such determination and focus when everything looks completely hopeless?

The challenges we face in life will not only be health challenges. At some point we will all likely face major health issues, and many will face other difficulties before a health crisis. All throughout our lives we will face difficult situations that may be social in nature, such as family relationships, cohabitation, marital, or partnership issues. Challenges may also surface in the form of a financial crisis or even a legal situation. When one is hit by one of these challenges, the real test is how one reacts and what course of action is taken. When one looks at immense scandalous challenges that seem to be repeatedly faced by so many political figures, it is worth noting the ones who survive are those who take time to analyze a given situation and consider the options before reacting. My brother Billy, a successful attorney, has said on more than one occasion, "If you are ever arrested for something, don't say anything." This is wise advice because when you say something in that situation, you unnecessarily make a commitment. It is better to be calm and remain silent, then approach the situation at a later time with an attorney who specializes in making good decisions in bad situations.

After the Vietnam War ended, I read a news article illustrating how the North Vietnamese soldiers were finding it difficult to accept life after war. During the war the soldiers were on a passionate mission and they happily accepted inhospitable living conditions and survived on meager rations. After the war was over, they became discontent with everything from their housing to their meals. I am able to relate because in many ways I have become a soldier without a war – or a rebel without a cause. Hence my newest goal is to prove James Schlesinger wrong by demonstrating there is more to this one American than just complacency and panic.

John F. Kennedy said that the decision to land a man on the moon and return him safely to the earth within the already tumultuous decade of the 1960s was made *because* it was no easy feat. He said that the United States would accomplish this goal simply because it was a challenge the American people were willing to accept, one on which they would waste no time, and one that they would win.

A strong determination to live is deeply ingrained in all of us. We have heard stories of people who perform heroic acts of strength during desperate situations. I remember my 5th grade teacher telling our class about a woman who hit a child with her car. When she exited the vehicle and saw the boy trapped under the car, she acted without thinking and *lifted the car* to free the boy. This story stuck in my mind and what I find remarkable is that here, an ordinary person was able to accomplish a truly astonishing feat having never even practiced weightlifting. I strongly believe we are all capable of doing things that are commonly accepted as impossible. The question is how far we are willing to go to accomplish such feats. In my particular case it was a matter of choice. The easy choice would have been to take the permanent disability and have my needs provided for from that point forward. The difficult part was to reject 'the easy choice' and travel the road less taken.

After considering what life would be like on permanent disability, I decided there was no other option. Like Nando Parrado, I saw no salvation beyond an expanse of snow-capped mountains. There was no obvious reason to continue, but I refused to accept what was before my eyes. I made the same decision to keep pushing forward as far as I could, knowing that it would not be easy.

The more I have studied those who have accomplished the remarkable, the less I believe in true genius. Johann Sebastian Bach may be considered a genius, but in my mind, his inhuman legacy has more to do with his industriousness than his inherent talent. This is why I believe each and every one of us is capable of doing such extraordinary things. Admittedly I am not a genius in any sense. When I was in middle-school, my poor grades were a reflection of how little I applied myself. I spent more time watching television than I did reading, and for that I paid the price. In 11th grade when I took the SAT, my score was embarrassingly low. Those paltry academic results stemmed from unwillingness and an inability to focus on the subjects that failed to hold my interest. My success on the cello may seem impressive, but I attribute it to working harder and putting in more effort than most. If I have been blessed with some gift, it is the ability to persevere. I have not as such been blessed with any inherent "genius" talent. I was however able to beat an incurable illness and therefore I am convinced that anyone is capable of doing the same.

I did not have a book as a guide, or guidance from any one individual in particular. My own accomplishments grew out of desperate determination. Accepting an MS-determined course on the downslope was not a possibility in my mind. There was never any premonition that I would face a life-threatening illness, and I had no idea what I was capable of under such circumstances. We are all capable of more than we realize and it often takes such a desperate situation to bring out the invincible fighter in each of us.

When diagnosed with a disease that may seem totally hopeless, consider what I have done. I am a professional musician with no background in science or medicine. My only knowledge of these subjects comes from a basic class I took in high school. Most of my life has been devoted to the cello. I had limited knowledge and resources to work with when fighting this disease; it was on-the-job training and I learned as I went. For others to successfully battle MS, I have set forth this guidebook from which everyone can learn and develop their own strategies for dealing with any challenge. When I was diagnosed with MS, I was desperate for some kind of detailed guide written by someone who had beaten the disease. Writing and assembling such a guide has been a long and difficult journey, but nothing in life that is worthwhile comes easily. The baton is now passed on to others so that they may also fight and conquer.

"I worked hard. Anyone who works as hard as I did can achieve the same results." - Johann Sebastian Bach

Appendix – Sources Cited

The web sources listed below are accessible as of February, 2016.

1. "Definition of MS." National Multiple Sclerosis Society. Web.
2. "Early Symptoms of Multiple Sclerosis (MS): Tingling, Numbness, Balance, and More." WebMD. Web.
3. "Effects of MS." Healthline. Web.
4. "How Does Heat Intolerance Affect Multiple Sclerosis?" About.com Health. Web.
5. "Lhermitte's Sign (and MS): What It Is and How to Treat It." Healthline. Web.
6. "Multiple Sclerosis Incontinence Treatment: Bladder Control Problems and More." WebMD. Web.
7. "Neurogenic Bladder: MedlinePlus Medical Encyclopedia." U.S National Library of Medicine. Web.
8. "PDUFA Legislation and Background." Prescription Drug User Fee Act. U.S. Food and Drug Administration, 2015. Web. http://www.fda.gov/ForIndustry/UserFees/PrescriptionDrugUserFee/ucm144411.htm
9. "Survival." U.S. Army Field Manual 3-05.70: SURVIVAL. 2002. United States Government – Department of the Army. Print.
10. "The MS Hug: What Is It? How Is It Treated?" Healthline. Web.
11. "Atlas, Multiple Sclerosis Resources in the World." World Health Organization. World Health Organization, 2008. Web. http://www.who.int/mental_health/neurology/Atlas_MS_WEB.pdf
12. "PDUFA Legislation and Background." US Food and Drug Administration.
13. Applebaum, Samuel and Applebaum, Sada. "Jascha Heifetz" *The Way They Play.* 1st ed. Vol. 1. Neptune City, NJ: Paganiniana Publications, 1972. 61-82. Print
14. Auer, Leopold. *Violin Playing as I Teach It.* New York: Frederick A. Stokes, 1921. Print.
15. Batmanghelidj F. "The Water Cure" Web. http://www.watercure.com
16. Batmanghelidj F. *Your Body's Many Cries for Water.* Global Health Solutions, Inc. 1997. Print.

17. Brzycki, Matt. *A Practical Approach to Strength Training.* Rev. ed. Grand Rapids, Mich.: Masters, 1991. Print.

18. Rogaine– Application Number NPA 20-834 http://www.accessdata.fda.gov/drugsatfda_docs/nda/97/20834_ROG AINE%20EXTRA%20STRENGTH%20FOR%20MEN%205%25_M EDR.PDF

19. Fischer, Bobby. *My 60 Memorable Games.* Bobby Fischer, 1969. Simon and Schuster. Print.

20. Fontana L. The Scientific Basis of Caloric Restriction Leading to Longer Life. *Current Opinion in Gastroenterology.* 2009;25(2):144-50. Print.

21. Nester, Tony. *Desert Survival Tips, Tricks, and Skills.* 2003. Diamond Creek Press. Print.

22. Grandjean AC, Reimers KJ, Bannick KE, and Haven MC. The Effect of Caffeinated, Non-Caffeinated, Caloric and Non-Caloric Beverages on Hydration. *Journal of the American College of Nutrition*; 2000; 19(5):591-600. Print.

23. Grandjean AC, Campbell SM. Water requirements, impinging factors and recommended intakes. *ILSI North America, Hydration: Fluids for Life* (2004). Web.

24. Hafler D. Multiple Sclerosis. *Journal of Clinical Investigation.* American Society for Clinical Investigation. Web. 2004;113(6):788-94.

25. Hinninghofen H and Enck P. Passenger Well-being in Airplanes. *Autonomic Neuroscience.* 2006; 1(1-2):80-85. Print.

26. Jacobs LD, Cookfair DL, Rudick RA, et al. Intramuscular interferon beta-1a for disease progression in relapsing multiple sclerosis. *Annals of Neurology.* 1996;39(3):285-94

27. Jacobs LD, Beck RW, Simon JH, et al. Intramuscular interferon beta-1a initiated during a first demyelinating event in multiple sclerosis. *New England Journal of Medicine.* 2000; 343(13):898-904.

28. Ketelhut R. "Physical Activity in Spite of Chronic Diseases." *The American Journal of Medicine and Sports.* 1999; 293-204. Print.

29. Kurtzke JF. Rating neurologic impairment in multiple sclerosis: an expanded disability status scale (EDSS). *Neurology.* 1983;33:1444-1452.

30. Parrado, Nando and Rause, Vince. *Miracle in the Andes: 72 Days on the Mountain and My Long Trek Home.* New York: Crown, 2006. Print.

31. Ryan, Nolan and House, Tom. *Nolan Ryan's Pitcher's Bible: The Ultimate Guide to Power, Precision, and Long-term Performance.* New York: Simon & Schuster, 1991. Print.

32. Silva, Jose and Stone, Robert B. *You the Healer: The World-famous Silva Method on How to Heal Yourself and Others.* Novato, Calif.: New World Library, 2005. Print.

33. Suzuki M, Wilcox B, and Wilcox C. "Okinawa Centenarian Study." Okinawa Centenarian Study. Web. http://www.okicent.org/study.html

34. Vishnudevananda, Swami. *The Complete Illustrated Book of Yoga.* New York: Three Rivers, 1988. Print.

35. http://www.whfoods.com/genpage.php?tname=foodspice&dbid=57#healthbenefits

36. https://www.organicfacts.net/health-benefits/fruit/health-benefits-of-raisins.html

37. http://www.mayoclinic.org/diseases-conditions/heart-disease/in-dcpth/nuts/art-20046635

38. http://www.medicalnewstoday.com/articles/269468.php

39. https://www.organicfacts.net/health-benefits/seed-and-nut/health-benefits-of-pistachio.html

40. http://www.medicaldaily.com/health-benefits-blueberries-5-reasons-eat-more-blueberries-246727

41. http://www.philly.com/philly/health/10_health_benefits_of_blueberries.html

42. http://www.arthritistoday.org/what-you-can-do/eating-well/benefits-of-eating-well/berries-benefits.php

43. http://berryhealth.fst.oregonstate.edu/health_healing/fact_sheets/

44. http://www.mcdicalnewstoday.com/articles/267290.php

45. http://healthyeating.sfgate.com/importance-eating-bananas-4466.html

46. http://www.medicalnewstoday.com/articles/276903.php

47. http://www.webmd.com/diet/8-healthy-facts-about-grapes

48. http://www.medicalnewstoday.com/articles/271156.php

49. http://www.webmd.com/food-recipes/all-about-avocados

50. http://www.whfoods.com/genpage.php?tname=foodspice&dbid=104

51. http://www.nutrition-and-you.com/watercress.html

52. http://www.cdc.gov/pcd/issues/2014/13_0390.htm
53. http://www.watercress.com/pdf/pot_health_benefits_of_wc_09.pdf
54. http://www.symptomfind.com/nutrition-supplements/brown-rice-health-benefits/
55. http://www.vegkitchen.com/tips/10-reasons-why-brown-rice-is-the-healthy-choice/
56. http://www.medicalnewstoday.com/articles/274745.php
57. http://www.bbcgoodfood.com/howto/guide/health-benefits-quinoa
58. http://www.whfoods.com/genpage.php?tname=foodspice&dbid=79
59. http://www.bbcgoodfood.com/howto/guide/ingredient-focus-soya
60. http://www.medicalnewstoday.com/articles/278340.php
61. http://www.whfoods.com/genpage.php?tname=foodspice&dbid=126
62. http://www.fatsecret.com/Diary.aspx?pa=fjrd&rid=1857598
63. http://www.webmd.com/food-recipes/5-winter-superfoods-sweet-potatoes-nutrient-profile
64. http://www.medicalnewstoday.com/articles/281438.php
65. http://www.mayoclinic.org/diseases-conditions/heart-disease/in-depth/omega-3/art-20045614
66. http://www.whfoods.com/genpage.php?tname=foodspice&dbid=56
67. http://www.nutrition-and-you.com/green-peas.html
68. http://www.medicalnewstoday.com/articles/265990.php
69. http://www.webmd.com/vitamins-supplements/ingredientmono-961-ginger.aspx?activeingredientid=961&activeingredientname=ginger

Notes

Notes

Notes

Notes

Notes

Notes